Self-assessment in
Accident and Emergency Medicine

In memory of
'Tony' Cross OBE MD FRCS

Self-assessment in Accident and Emergency Medicine

Derek Burke FRCS (A&E) Ed
Accident and Emergency Department, The Manor
Hospital, Walsall Hospitals NHS Trust, UK

Ian Greaves MB ChB MRCP(UK) DTM&H DipIMC
Accident and Emergency Department, St James
University Hospital, Leeds, UK

Philip Hormbrey MB ChB MRCP(UK) DA DipIMC FRCS (A&E) Ed
Accident and Emergency Department, The Oxford
Radcliffe Hospital, UK

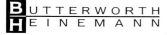

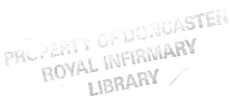

Butterworth-Heinemann
Linacre House, Jordan Hill, Oxford OX2 8DP
A division of Reed Educational and Professional Publishing Ltd

℞ A member of the Reed Elsevier plc group

OXFORD   BOSTON   JOHANNESBURG
MELBOURNE   NEW DELHI   SINGAPORE

First published 1996

British Library Cataloguing in Publication Data
A catalogue record for this book is available from the British Library

Library of Congress Cataloguing in Publication Data
A catalogue record for this book is available from the Library of Congress

ISBN 0 7506 2215 6

Composition by Genesis Typesetting, Laser Quay, Rochester, Kent
Printed in Great Britain at the University Press, Cambridge

Contents

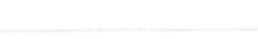

Foreword

It is a great pleasure, indeed an honour, to write the Foreword for this text.

Accident and Emergency Medicine is a young, but flourishing specialty. It follows, therefore, that there is a relative paucity of quality texts to guide the trainee, as well as the Consultant. Training in Emergency Medicine is now well established at both Registrar and Senior Registrar level, and Post-Calman trainees will enjoy a well-structured five year programme.

The second tier examination of the Royal College of Surgeons of Edinburgh (FRCS Ed. [A&E]) is now established as an enviable qualification but soon the exit fellowship of the Faculty of Accident and Emergency Medicine will be required at the end of training.

This text will be of great value to those preparing for both the FRCS (Ed. [A&E]) and the FFAEM, as well as those wishing to keep on top of current thinking. Not only is the reader stretched by the testing MCQ's, case histories, data interpretation, and clinical questions, but learns further by reviewing the well explained answers. This is an educationally sound learning method which uses scant available study time to the best advantage.

The authors are to be congratulated. The readers will be grateful, and as a result patient care 'in the front line' of clinical practice will improve.

David V. Skinner FFAEM, FRCS
Accident and Emergency Consultant

Preface

Accident and emergency (A&E) medicine by its very nature covers a very extensive field of study. The new senior house officer, perhaps only qualified for a year, can find the range of conditions presenting to the department quite daunting. With experience comes recognition of the common patterns of illness and injury and appreciation of situations where a more cautious clinical approach may be necessary. In this book we have aimed to outline the diagnosis and management of the common clinical situations in emergency medicine. We have used the format of multiple choice questions, case histories, data interpretations and picture questions as used in many of the postgraduate exams. Also included are the conditions that frequently result in medicolegal action, conditions where management remains contentious and the occasional rarity which may be seen from time to time in a busy department.

We hope the book will be used both by trainees wishing to pursue a career in emergency medicine who are studying for exams such as the FRCS(Ed) in A&E and the FFAEM, and also by recently qualified SHOs starting their first post in the specialty. We would be interested to hear of any suggestions or changes that could be made for future editions.

Derek Burke, Ian Greaves, Philip Hormbrey
Oxford, May 1995

Acknowledgements

We would like to thank our colleagues Fionna Moore, Stephen Miles and Clive Weston for inspiration, advice on medical education and help with providing the questions.

MULTIPLE CHOICE QUESTIONS

Trauma and orthopaedics

General

Q1 Regarding the Salter–Harris classification of fractures.

a Type II is the commonest.
b Type III involves both the epiphysis and metaphysis.
c Type V involves only the epiphysis.
d Slipped upper femoral epiphysis is a type I injury.
e Bennett's fracture in a 22-year-old man is a type II injury.

Q2 Sudeck's atrophy:

a May be treated by guanethidine block.
b Produces the radiological appearances of osteoporosis.
c Is most common after Colles fracture.
d Is not a complication of scaphoid fracture.
e Usually resolves within 12 months.

Q3 The following are true of compartment syndromes:

a Prolongation of capillary refill time is an early sign.
b They may be a complication of a bleeding disorder.
c The diagnosis may be confirmed by direct measurement of compartment pressure.
d Deep peroneal nerve palsy results from increased pressure in the posterior compartment of the calf.
e They may follow prolonged exercise.

Multiple choice questions

Q4 The following fractures and nerve injuries are associated:

a Anterior dislocation of the shoulder and axillary nerve palsy.
b Fractures of the shaft of the humerus and median nerve palsy.
c Supracondylar fracture of the humerus and median nerve palsy.
d Dislocation of the knee and common peroneal nerve palsy.
e Dislocation of the hip and sciatic nerve palsy.

Q5 Regarding a single eighth rib fracture in a patient with chronic obstructive airways disease:

a A chest X-ray should be performed.
b Prophylactic antibiotics should be prescribed.
c Strapping of the chest wall improves outcome.
d Symptoms usually resolve within 2 weeks.
e Oblique chest films should be performed.

Q6 Concerning hand infections:

a Septic arthritis is more common in the interphalangeal joints than in the metacarpophalangeal joints.
b Tendon sheath infections are characterized by exquisite pain on passive flexion.
c Paronychia are frequently caused by *Staphylococcus aureus*.
d Paronychia always require surgical drainage.
e Herpetic whitlows are caused by direct inoculation of the virus onto the distal finger.

Q7 Regarding the technique of haematoma block:

a It should not be used for a compound fracture.
b When used for a Colles fracture the approach should be from the volar aspect.
c Osteomyelitis occurs in 1% of cases.
d A venous tourniquet should be used to achieve maximal effectiveness.
e It can be used to reduce a metacarpal fracture.

2

Q8 In Bier's blockade:

a Bupivacaine should be used.
b The cuff should be inflated to the systolic blood pressure.
c A cannula should be placed in both arms.
d The cuff may be deflated as soon as the manipulation has taken place.
e Cardiovascular collapse is usually the first symptom of toxicity.

Q9 Regarding the Revised Trauma Score (RTS).

a Weighted values for pulse rate are used.
b A value of 7.84 is normal.
c It is a good triage tool for detecting victims of major trauma.
d The worst value in the first 24 hours after admission is used in the Major Trauma Outcome Study, (MTOS).
e It utilizes capillary refilling time.

Q10 Regarding the Glasgow Coma Score.

a The range of possible scores is 0–15.
b A score of 7 indicates coma.
c There are six possible verbal responses.
d Motor response to pain is assessed by pressing over the supraorbital nerve.
e An eye score of 2 indicates eye opening to speech.

Q11 Greenstick fractures:

a Usually require manipulation under general anaesthetic.
b Are otherwise known as torus fractures.
c Occur when only one side of the cortex is fractured.
d Are rarely angulated.
e Are usually epiphyseal.

Multiple choice questions

The upper limb

Q12 Regarding shoulder injuries:

a Frozen shoulder is commoner in the over-60s than the under-60s.
b Acromioclavicular dislocation requires percutaneous fixation.
c Fractured clavicle should be treated in a collar and cuff.
d Complete rotator cuff tears are best treated conservatively.
e Painful arc syndrome is characterized by pain when abducting between 0 and 60°.

Q13 Regarding dislocation of the shoulder:

a Posterior dislocation is a complication of epileptic fits.
b An anteroposterior view of the shoulder will clearly reveal posterior dislocations.
c Anterior dislocation is associated with the Bankhart lesion.
d Reduction usually requires general anaesthesia.
e Paraesthesia over the tip of the shoulder indicates axillary nerve palsy.

Q14 Regarding nerve injuries:

a The ulnar nerve is most vulnerable to injury at the elbow.
b Ulnar nerve injury results in weak adduction of the thumb.
c Median nerve injury causes wasting of the hypothenar eminence.
d Injury to the median nerve causes weak opposition of the thumb.
e Radial nerve palsy may cause wrist drop.

Q15 Concerning soft tissue conditions of the elbow:

a Golfer's elbow occurs at the common extensor origin.
b Chronic olecranon bursitis may require surgical treatment.
c Olecranon bursitis may require oral antibiotic treatment.
d Pain on shaking hands or opening doors is characteristic of tennis elbow.
e Haemarthrosis of the elbow in the absence of a fracture on the X-ray should be treated by early mobilization.

Q16 A fractured radial head:

a Is often caused by a fall on to an outstretched hand.
b Causes pain worsened by pronation and supination.
c Is a commonly missed diagnosis by junior doctors in the A&E department.
d Is a contraindication to joint aspiration.
e Leads to a residual loss of 10° of extension at the elbow in many cases.

Q17 Regarding elbow injuries:

a Pulled elbow has a characteristic radiological appearance.
b A raised anterior fat pad indicates an elbow effusion.
c Myositis ossificans is a complication of prolonged immobilization of an elbow haemarthrosis.
d Backward tilt of more than 15° is an indication for reduction of a supracondylar fracture.
e Undisplaced fracture of the olecranon is treated in a collar and cuff.

Q18 Concerning forearm fractures:

a Monteggia fracture–dislocation is associated with distal radioulnar dislocation.
b Galeazzi fracture–dislocation is associated with fracture of the distal radius.
c Median nerve palsy is a complication of missed Monteggia fractures.
d Compartment syndrome may complicate treatment of a Monteggia fracture.
e Isolated radial fracture can occur in the absence of radioulnar subluxation.

Q19 Colles fracture:

a Usually requires reduction if there is more than 10° of dorsal angulation.
b Is associated with the development of Sudeck's atrophy.
c Can be reduced using an axillary nerve block.
d May be complicated by delayed rupture of flexor pollicis longus.
e Is associated with an increased incidence of carpal tunnel syndrome.

Multiple choice questions

Q20 Regarding injuries around the wrist:

a A Smith's fracture requires immobilization in an above-elbow plaster.
b Scaphoid fracture can be excluded by normal scaphoid views 2 weeks following injury.
c Lunate dislocation is associated with ulnar nerve compression.
d Fracture of the radial styloid requires immobilization in a Colles plaster for 6 weeks.
e Barton's fracture is a type of Colles fracture in which only the dorsal part of the radius is involved.

Q21 Regarding scaphoid fractures.

a Tenderness in the anatomical snuffbox is diagnostic.
b Distal fractures are more common than proximal fractures.
c Avascular necrosis complicates 30% of distal pole fractures.
d Avascular necrosis is usually evident on X-rays at 2 weeks.
e Immobilizing plaster should include the interphalangeal joint of the thumb.

Q22 Tenosynovitis at the wrist:

a Is an occupational hazard of keyboard operators.
b May be treated in a scaphoid plaster.
c Produces a positive Finkelstein's test.
d Most commonly occurs in the tendon of flexor carpi radialis.
e May respond to steroid injection.

Q23 Carpal dislocation:

a May result from a fall on an outstretched hand.
b Is most commonly an isolated lunate dislocation.
c May be associated with scaphoid fracture.
d Is associated with median nerve palsy.
e Is usually dorsal.

Q24 Carpal tunnel syndrome:

a Classically produces pain and paraesthesiae at night.
b Responds to oral steroid therapy.
c Is associated with pregnancy.
d May result in wrist drop.
e Is eight times more common in women than men.

Q25 The ulnar collateral ligament of the thumb:

a Is often injured in skiing accidents.
b If ruptured should be treated by strapping and early mobilization.
c If torn compromises the ability to extend the thumb.
d Is more commonly ruptured than the radial collateral ligament.
e When torn should be repaired in the A&E department.

Q26 Regarding hand injuries:

a Bennett's fracture is frequently associated with ulnar collateral ligament injury at the metacarpophalangeal joint.
b Bennett's fracture can be managed by closed manipulation and immobilization in plaster.
c Fractures of the fifth metacarpal may result in extensor lag.
d Clenched fist injuries rarely involve the metacarpophalangeal joint.
e Up to 15° of rotational deformity is acceptable in a proximal phalanx fracture.

Q27 Regarding tendon injuries:

a Division of flexor digitorum profundus results in loss of flexion at the proximal interphalangeal joint.
b Division of an extensor tendon leads to complete loss of extension at the metacarpophalangeal joint.
c Rupture of the middle slip of flexor digitorum superficialis leads to a swan neck deformity.
d Ruptured flexor tendons should be repaired in A&E.
e Repaired extensor tendons should be immobilized with the metacarpophalangeal joints in 180° of extension.

Q28 Regarding finger injuries:

a A mallet finger should be treated in a mallet splint for 2 weeks.
b Minor sprains of the proximal interphalangeal joints should be treated with a period of immobilization of 5 days.
c Neighbour strapping can be used to manage minor finger sprains.
d A Bedford splint can be used to manage minor finger sprains.
e The prognosis of distal interphalangeal joint injuries tends to be worse than those of the proximal interphalangeal joint.

Multiple choice questions

Pelvis and lower limb

Q29 Regarding pelvic fractures:

a Bucket-handle fractures have the highest mortality.
b There may be no signs on initial clinical assessment.
c Springing the pelvis is a useful diagnostic test.
d There is an increased risk of small-bowel injury.
e Pelvic fracture may be associated with massive blood loss.

Q30 Posterior dislocation of the hip:

a Accounts for 20% of hip dislocations.
b Is associated with loss of dorsiflexion of the foot.
c Causes flexion and external rotation of the leg.
d Usually requires general anaesthesia for reduction.
e Requires admission for rest and traction.

Q31 Concerning hip conditions in children:

a Perthes disease is twice as common in boys.
b Slipped upper femoral epiphysis has a peak incidence at 4–8 years of age.
c Perthes disease is commoner in fat, hypogonadal children.
d Treatment of slipped upper femoral epiphysis is surgical.
e Transient synovitis may mimic Perthes disease and slipped upper femoral epiphysis.

Q32 Fractured neck of femur:

a Presents with shortening and internal rotation of the leg.
b May be complicated by avascular necrosis.
c May present several weeks after a fall.
d Commonly presents with bruising over the greater trochanter.
e Under the age of 60 is commoner in men.

Q33 Fractures of the femoral shaft:

a Are associated with pelvic fractures.
b If closed usually result in approximately 2 litres of blood loss.
c Can be immobilized in a traction splint.
d Are associated with fat embolism.
e Are often pathological over the age of 50.

Q34 Regarding knee injuries:

a The lateral collateral ligament is the most frequently damaged ligament.
b An effusion immediately following an injury indicates the presence of a haemarthrosis.
c Anterior cruciate injuries result in difficulty in walking upstairs.
d Tenderness over the joint line indicates a collateral ligament injury.
e Tense haemarthroses should be aspirated.

Q35 The following conditions can cause knee pain in children:

a Osgood–Schlatter disease.
b Chondromalacia patellae.
c Perthes disease.
d Rheumatoid arthritis.
e Henoch–Schönlein purpura.

Q36 Concerning fractures of the lower leg:

a Compound fractures constitute 50% of all fractures.
b Undisplaced tibial fractures in children are treated in a long leg plaster.
c The popliteal artery may be damaged in upper tibial fractures.
d Avascular necrosis of the proximal tibial fragment may occur.
e Anterior shin pain in an athlete may suggest stress fracture of the tibia.

Q37 Achilles tendon rupture:

a Is most common in middle-aged men.
b Usually occurs at the site of insertion of the tendon.
c Can be precipitated by local steroid injections.
d Leads to inability to dorsiflex the foot against opposition.
e Can be treated in an equinus plaster.

Multiple choice questions

Q38 Regarding ankle injuries:

a Most result from an eversion sprain.
b A simple sprain should resolve within 10 days.
c Dislocation at the ankle mortice should be reduced under general anaesthetic in theatre.
d A fractured fibula above the distal tibiofibular joint requires internal fixation.
e The Maisonneuve fracture is a fracture of the medial malleolus associated with a fracture of the proximal tibia.

Q39 Fractures of the calcaneum :

a Are usually caused in road traffic accidents.
b Are associated with fractures at the dorsolumbar junction.
c May cause a decrease in Böhler's angle.
d Are associated with central dislocation of the hip.
e Involving the subtalar joint commonly result in secondary osteoarthritis.

Q40 Regarding foot injuries:

a Undisplaced metatarsal fractures must be treated with a walking plaster.
b A March fracture involves the second or third proximal phalanx.
c The Jones fracture is a fracture of the fifth metatarsal.
d Avulsion fracture of the first metatarsal is the commonest fracture of the foot.
e Fractures of the talar neck classically occur in aircraft accidents.

Head and spine

Q41 The following are characteristic of base of skull fracture:

a Fluid level in frontal sinus on skull X-ray.
b Tympanic membrane tear.
c Otorrhoea.
d Infraorbital nerve paraesthesia.
e Subhyaloid haemorrhage.

Q42 Regarding skull fracture:

a A double shadow on an X-ray indicates a depressed fracture.
b Palpation of scalp lacerations will reveal fractures not visible on X-ray.
c Require 6 months for complete radiological resolution.
d Computed tomographic (CT) scan reveals more fractures than standard skull views.
e Fluid in the sphenoid sinus suggests basal fracture.

Q43 The following are indications for skull X-ray of an adult with a head injury:

a 5 cm laceration to the vertex.
b Loss of consciousness.
c Persistent vomiting.
d Forehead haematoma.
e Patient drunk.

Q44 Indications for neurosurgical referral in head injury include:

a Pinpoint pupils.
b Generalized convulsions.
c Amnesia.
d Cranial vault fracture.
e Persistent vomiting.

Q45 Mannitol in head injury:

a May be indicated when definitive treatment is likely to be delayed.
b Should only be given after discussion with a neurosurgeon.
c Is given at a dose of 1 g/kg of a 50% solution.
d May cause intracranial pressure to rise.
e May cause systemic hypotension.

Q46 Regarding whiplash injuries:

a Symptoms usually resolve within 2 weeks of injury.
b Cervical X-rays are mandatory.
c The central cord syndrome is commoner in the under-50s.
d They predispose to early cervical spondylosis.
e They should be treated by the use of a soft collar for 2 weeks.

Multiple choice questions

Q47 Concerning spinal cord injuries:

a Hypotension can be adequately corrected with fluids.
b Bradycardia does not respond to atropine.
c Priapism is common.
d Cervical collar adequately immobilizes the cervical spine.
e The maximum neurological deficit is usually seen immediately following blunt trauma.

Q48 Regarding spinal fractures:

a Fractures are more common at C7/T1 and T12/L1 than in the mid thoracic zone.
b Thoracic fractures are more common in women than men.
c Patients should be catheterized in the A&E department.
d Jefferson's fracture describes a fracture of the axis (C2).
e Vertebral subluxation of 33% suggests a unilateral facet dislocation.

Q49 Regarding cervical spine injury:

a The neck should be immobilized in the position in which it was found.
b Type I odontoid fractures are usually stable.
c Type III odontoid fractures occur through the tip of the peg.
d The 'hangman's' fracture is a fracture of the atlas.
e Neurological deficit in the absence of a fracture is rare.

Q50 Concerning cervical spine radiography:

a Apparent subluxation of C3 on C4 may be a normal appearance in infants.
b Significant injury is excluded by a normal lateral cervical spine film.
c Three views should be requested.
d A 'swimmer's' view may be required for adequate visualization of the cervical spine.
e In an adult a distance of more than 3 mm from the anterior arch of C1 to the anterior edge of the odontoid is abnormal.

Maxillofacial injuries

Q51 Laryngeal fractures are associated with:

a Hoarseness.
b Haemoptysis.
c Subcutaneous emphysema of the neck.
d Fracture of the hyoid bone.
e Cervical spine injury.

Q52 A 'blow-out' orbital fracture may be associated with:

a Diplopia.
b Infraorbital nerve paraesthesia.
c Hyphaema.
d Subcutaneous emphysema of the upper lid.
e The 'teardrop' sign on X-ray.

Q53 Concerning nasal fractures:

a Early X-rays are essential for management.
b Septal haematoma is managed conservatively.
c Septal deviation is an indication for reduction.
d Cerebrospinal fluid rhinorrhoea may indicate a nasoethmoid fracture.
e Antibiotic cover is required.

Q54 Regarding the mandible:

a Fractures are best seen on standard anteroposterior and lateral X-rays.
b Fractures are usually single.
c Dislocations can be caused by yawning.
d Dislocations are always bilateral.
e Dislocations are associated with a closed mouth.

Q55 Following trauma, loose teeth:

a Have a 50% chance of survival if reimplanted.
b Can be kept between the gum and the cheek.
c Should be retained in a container of formalin.
d May be aspirated.
e Should be wired back in place in the A&E department.

Multiple choice questions

Trauma resuscitation

Q56 Regarding the management of major trauma (Advanced Trauma Life Support; ATLS):

a The first priority is gaining venous access.
b Central lines are preferable to peripheral lines for resuscitation.
c Supplemental oxygen should only be given when hypoxia has been demonstrated.
d Cervical collars can be removed when normal cervical spine X-rays have been obtained.
e Failure to visualize C7/T1 on standard lateral views indicates the need for CT scan.

Q57 Regarding open chest injuries:

a A defect of more than two-thirds of the tracheal diameter leads to preferential air flow through the defect.
b An occlusive dressing sealed to the chest wall on all four sides should be used.
c A chest drain should be inserted through the wound.
d Surgical repair is always required.
e A prophylactic chest drain on the contralateral side is required in all cases.

Q58 Regarding tension pneumothorax:

a The trachea is shifted to the side of the pneumothorax.
b An immediate portable chest X-ray should be performed prior to drainage.
c The neck veins may be distended.
d It must be treated initially with an intercostal drain.
e It is a complication of subclavian line insertion.

Q59 Cardiac tamponade:

a Is usually characterized by the presence of over 100 ml of blood in the pericardial sac.
b Is associated with distended neck veins.
c Is characterized by hypertension.
d Must be treated by immediate thoracotomy.
e Is often diagnosed late.

Q60 Myocardial contusion is characterized by:

a Raised cardiac enzymes.
b Sinus bradycardia.
c Multiple premature ventricular beats.
d ST depression.
e Right bundle branch block.

Q61 Concerning needle cricothyroidotomy:

a It is contraindicated in the under-12s.
b The cricoid membrane lies immediately below the cricoid cartilage.
c It provides adequate ventilation for 45 minutes.
d It is preferable to minitracheostomy in the acute situation.
e It may be complicated by oesophageal perforation.

Q62 Regarding diagnostic peritoneal lavage:

a It is absolutely contraindicated in cirrhosis.
b It is 75% sensitive for intraperitoneal bleeding.
c It is positive if the effluent fluid contains greater than 100 000 red blood cells per cubic millilitre.
d It may produce a false positive result in a patient with pelvic fractures.
e It is indicated in patients with signs of peritoneal irritation after major trauma.

Q63 Regarding diagnostic peritoneal lavage:

a A bladder catheter should be inserted.
b A nasogastric tube is not required.
c A midline upper abdominal approach should be used.
d Greater than 5000 leukocytes per cubic millimetre indicates the need for laparotomy.
e A negative result excludes intra abdominal pathology.

Multiple choice questions

Q64 Regarding injury to the genitourinary tract:

a It can be excluded if the patient does not have haematuria.
b The volume of blood in the urine correlates well with the severity of the trauma.
c 50% of renal injuries will need operative intervention.
d The urinary bladder is more prone to injury when full than when empty.
e If urethral injury is suspected, a retrograde urethrogram should be performed.

Q65 Cranial CT in major trauma:

a Will exclude odontoid peg fractures.
b Eliminates the need for plain skull radiographs.
c Should be performed with contrast.
d Will demonstrate cerebral contusion.
e Distinguishes extradural and subdural bleeding.

Q66 Retroperitoneal haemorrhage:

a May be from the pancreas.
b May be detected on peritoneal lavage.
c May obscure the psoas shadow on plain abdominal X-ray.
d May be suggested by fractures of the spinous processes on X-ray.
e May be associated with periumbilical bruising.

Q67 Concerning urological trauma:

a It is more common in men than women.
b Posterior urethral injuries occur in up to 40% of pelvic fractures.
c Significant injury is commonly revealed by the presence of microscopic haematuria.
d Blood at the meatus indicates the need for retrograde urethrography.
e In women it can be associated with vaginal bleeding.

Medicine

General and Cardiology

Q68 In acute myocardial infarction thrombolysis is contraindicated:

a If the patient is pregnant.
b In the presence of active peptic ulceration.
c Within 6 months of a cerebrovascular haemorrhage.
d In patients on warfarin.
e Following central venous cannulation.

Q69 Myocardial infarction:

a Is the commonest cause of death in the UK.
b May produce a fever up to 38°C.
c Is associated with a peak creatinine kinase level at 48–72 hours.
d Is likely to be complicated by complete heart block in anterior infarction.
e May be associated with a normal electrocardiogram (ECG).

Q70 Cardiogenic shock after myocardial infarction:

a Causes hypotension, peripheral vasoconstriction and oliguria.
b Is associated with metabolic alkalosis.
c Is more common after an inferior rather than an anterior infarct.
d Is treated with sympathomimetics.
e Has a survival rate of 80% if treated early.

Q71 Regarding Addison's disease:

a Onset may be insidious.
b Infection may precipitate a crisis.
c Hydrocortisone alone is required for steroid replacement.
d Tuberculosis is the commonest cause.
e The diagnosis is suggested by a raised serum potassium and lowered serum sodium.

Multiple choice questions

Q72 Regarding hypoglycaemia:

a Intravenous glucose 50 ml of 50% is the treatment of choice in adults.
b A serum glucose level of 4 mmol/l excludes the diagnosis.
c It is a common finding in neonates.
d Resistant cases may require administration of IV dexamethasone.
e It may recur after treatment in patients on sulphonylureas.

Q73 In cases of hyperglycaemia:

a The vision may be blurred.
b Urine testing is not required if the serum glucose is less than 20 mmol/l.
c Hyperkalaemia should be treated with calcium resonium.
d Admission is mandatory.
e Blood glucose should be brought down to less than 5 mmol/l within 4 hours.

Q74 Regarding the 1993 British Thoracic Society's (BTS) guidelines for the management of asthma in the A&E department:

a Arterial blood gases are recommended for all patients with peak flow less than 50% predicted value.
b IV aminophylline is recommended for patients with peak flow less than 33%.
c A $Pao_2 < 8$ kPa and/or a $Paco_2 > 6$ kPa indicate respiratory failure.
d High flow oxygen (minimum 60%) should be given to all patients.
e A pulse ≥ 110 beats/min and/or respiratory rate ≥ 25 breaths/min indicate severe asthma.

Q75 Features suggesting organic headache include:

a Failure to respond to analgesics.
b Tight constricting pain.
c Scalp tenderness.
d Increasing severity with cough.
e Early morning headache.

Q76 Clinical features of temporal arteritis include:

a Ophthalmoplegia.
b Weight loss.
c Transient ischaemic attack.
d A raised erythrocyte sedimentation rate (ESR) in all cases.
e Pain on eating.

Q77 Acute gout:

a Is always associated with a raised serum uric acid.
b Is eight times more common in men than women.
c Can be diagnosed using polarized light microscopy.
d Should be treated with allopurinol.
e Responds to colchicine.

Q78 Migraine:

a Is five times as common in women as in men.
b Can be precipitated by monosodium glutamate.
c Is typically unilateral at onset.
d Is a cause of dysphasia.
e Should be treated with oral ergotamine.

Q79 Regarding hypothermia:

a Hypothermia is defined as a core temperature less than 36°C.
b Spontaneous ventricular fibrillation is likely to occur at a temperature of 30°C.
c Serum amylase should be measured.
d IV fluids should be administered.
e Passive warming is adequate in most cases.

Q80 Regarding crescendo angina:

a Aspirin should be prescribed.
b ST depression on ECG during attacks is a common finding.
c Cardiac enzymes are raised following an episode.
d The risk of myocardial infarction is the same as for normal angina.
e Admission is mandatory.

Multiple choice questions

Q81 Regarding pulmonary embolus:

a ECG signs of right heart strain is a common finding.
b Linear collapse on chest X-ray is characteristic.
c A coexisting clinically evident deep venous thrombosis (DVT) is likely to be found.
d A $Pao_2 < 10$ kPa is characteristically found in symptomatic embolus.
e V/Q scan is as sensitive as pulmonary arteriography in detecting clots.

Q82 Regarding epilepsy:

a Normal oxygen saturation during a fit suggests the diagnosis of pseudofit.
b Parenteral diazepam is the drug of choice to control acute fits.
c IV phenytoin should be administered under ECG control.
d Patients having a first fit should be admitted to hospital.
e Nocturnal fits are a contraindication to driving.

Q83 Regarding atypical chest pain:

a A normal ECG confidently excludes a diagnosis of myocardial infarction.
b Viral costochondritis is a common cause.
c A normal chest X-ray excludes pulmonary embolus.
d Right-sided chest pain is not associated with myocardial infarction.
e Urinalysis should always be performed.

Q84 Deep venous thrombosis:

a Can be excluded by ultrasonography.
b Produces a positive Homans sign.
c Is best detected by venography.
d Requires admission.
e May be treated by thrombolysis.

Q85 Transient ischaemic attacks (TIAs):

a Last less than 12 hours.
b May be associated with amnesia.
c May mimic migraine.
d Are caused by thromboembolism in 60% of cases.
e Lead to a completed stroke in 50% of patients at 5 years.

Q86 Concerning subarachnoid haemorrhage:

a Subhyaloid haemorrhage may be found.
b Nimodipine reduces the mortality.
c Results from 'berry' aneurysm in 95% of cases.
d Diagnosis is made by CT scan.
e It may be preceded by intermittent attacks of headache.

Q87 Concerning sickle cell anaemia:

a It is an autosomal dominant disease.
b A patient with known sickle cell disease who presents in crisis should have analgesia withheld until a definite diagnosis is made.
c Neurological complications are rare.
d Haemoglobin below 10 g/dl occurs in 10% of cases.
e An aplastic crisis can be induced by folate deficiency.

Resuscitation

Q88 Central venous cannulation:

a Should usually be performed on the left side of the neck.
b Is indicated for fluid administration in shock.
c By the subclavian route has a pneumothorax rate of 5% in the emergency situation.
d Allows right heart filling pressure to be monitored.
e Is most safely achieved by the subclavian route.

Q89 Regarding cardiac arrest:

a The gold standard for drug administration is the central route.
b Drugs can be delivered using an intraosseous technique.
c Opioid analgesics should be given early.
d All patients should be defibrillated prior to connection to a monitor.
e Resuscitation should stop if the pupils dilate.

Q90 In the treatment of electromechanical dissociation (EMD):

a Atropine 3 mg is given once.
b 10 ml calcium chloride should be given routinely.
c In children an IV fluid bolus is given.
d Adrenaline 5 mg may be considered if the arrest is prolonged.
e Pericardiocentesis may be attempted.

Multiple choice questions

Q91 In a monitored arrest secondary to ventricular fibrillation:

a A precordial thump may be of value.
b Synchronized cardioversion should be used.
c Adrenaline 10 ml 1:10 000 is the first drug that should be given.
d Atropine should be used as a second line drug.
e The prognosis is worse than in an asystolic arrest.

Q92 Asystolic cardiac arrrest:

a Cannot be diagnosed if 'p' waves are present.
b May respond to cardiac pacing if electrical activity is present.
c Is an indication for the use of adrenaline 1 mg.
d Is an indication for the use of atropine 3 mg.
e Is the commonest arrest rhythm in children.

Q93 Electromechanical dissociation:

a Means electrical activity with no cardiac output.
b Can be caused by β-blockers.
c May be caused by hypothermia.
d May be caused by ketamine.
e Should be treated with lignocaine.

Q94 The following are true:

a Lignocaine improves the response to defibrillation in ventricular fibrillation.
b Adenosine slows conduction through the atrioventricular node.
c Bretylium is effective in 2–5 minutes.
d Atropine antagonizes the action of acetylcholine at muscarinic receptors.
e Lignocaine is contraindicated in torsade de pointes.

Q95 Adrenaline:

a Should not be self-administered by a patient.
b Is not effective given by the endotracheal route.
c Increases the maximum safe dose of lignocaine that be given in a digital nerve block.
d Is given every 5 minutes in cardiac arrest.
e May be given intravenously in anaphylaxis.

Q96 Sodium bicarbonate:

a Contains 10 mmol bicarbonate in 10 ml 8.4% solution.
b Cannot be given with calcium.
c May exacerbate intracellular acidosis.
e Causes tissue ulceration.
e Should be used early in the course of cardiac arrest.

Q97 Laryngeal masks:

a Are the method of choice in advanced airway management in cardiac arrest.
b Provide as good protection against inhalation of stomach contents as an endotracheal tube.
c Can be used as an aid to endotracheal intubation.
d Are available in the same range of sizes as endotracheal tubes.
e Are reusable.

Q98 Regarding airway adjuncts:

a A size 3 Guedel airway would be suitable for an average adult.
b The nasopharyngeal airway stimulates the gag reflex less than the Guedel airway.
c The Laerdal pocket mask can only be used in adults.
d A size 4.5 endotracheal tube is suitable for a 3-year-old.
e Sellick's manoeuvre reduces the risk of aspiration in endotracheal intubation.

Q99 Open cardiac massage:

a May be indicated in penetrating cardiac trauma.
b Produces a higher cardiac output than closed cardiac massage.
c Is indicated in cardiac arrest in patients with emphysema.
d Should be performed via a median sternotomy.
e Has a survival rate to discharge of 70% in all patients.

Q100 When used in resuscitation, lignocaine:

a May be ineffective in hypothermia.
b Stabilizes membranes by impeding sodium transport.
c May be given by the endotracheal route.
d Should be used to treat electromechanical dissociation.
e Is indicated in the treatment of ventricular tachycardia.

Multiple choice questions

Q101 In distinguishing supraventricular tachycardia with aberrant conduction and ventricular tachycardia:

a Adenosine may be used.
b Atrioventricular dissociation indicates a supraventricular origin.
c Capture beats indicate a ventricular origin.
d A previous 12-lead ECG may be useful.
e Concordant QRS polarity in the chest leads indicates a ventricular origin.

Q102 Supraventricular tachycardia:

a Is associated with Wolff–Parkinson–White syndrome.
b Will respond to adenosine in over 90% of cases.
c Should be treated with verapamil if the patient has a low blood pressure.
d Is associated with caffeine intake.
e Can be terminated with adrenaline.

Q103 Regarding heart block:

a In a first-degree heart block the PR interval is more than 0.2 seconds.
b Type I second degree heart block is characterized by a constant PR interval.
c In third-degree heart block the RR interval is variable.
d In type II second degree heart block there are no missed beats.
e Type I second degree heart block is more likely to proceed to ventricular fibrillation than type II.

Q104 In complete heart block:

a The PR interval is constant.
b The heart rate is usually less than 60 beats/minute.
c Atropine may improve the rate.
d Pacing is usually required.
e Hypotension is a feature.

Overdose and substance abuse

Q105 Tricyclic antidepressant overdose may be complicated by:

a Convulsions.
b Coma.
c Urinary retention.
d Hepatic failure.
e Dry mouth.

Q106 Features of mefenamic acid (Ponstan) overdose include:

a Diarrhoea.
b Reduced conscious level.
c Convulsions.
d Cardiac arrhythmias.
e Acute renal failure.

Q107 Benzodiazepines:

a Require gastric lavage if taken in overdose.
b May cause hostile and aggressive behaviour.
c May cause tinnitus on withdrawal.
d May be treated with naloxone if taken in overdose.
e Are valuable in the management of chronic anxiety states.

Q108 Aspirin overdose:

a Presents as a metabolic acidosis in young children.
b Causes convulsions.
c May be treated by forced alkaline diuresis.
d Presents with a respiratory acidosis.
e May be treated with activated charcoal.

Q109 Overdose of co-proxamol:

a May require ventilation.
b Responds to naloxone.
c Is not usually clinically significant if the paracetamol levels are
   below the treatment threshold.
d Can lead to liver failure.
e Is potentiated by alcohol.

Multiple choice questions

Q110 Following a single acute episode of solvent abuse, clinical features may include:

a Coma.
b Ataxia.
c Renal failure.
d Cardiac arrest.
e Convulsions.

Q111 Concerning cannabis abuse:

a Symptoms characteristically last 6–12 hours following inhalation.
b Cough may occur.
c The ECG may be abnormal.
d Coma with dilated pupils may develop.
e Perception of colour can be enhanced.

Q112 Regarding alcohol abuse:

a The liver is normal in 80% of alcoholics.
b 10% of those with cirrhosis will progress to liver failure.
c Chlormethiazole (Heminevrin) may be used to control acute withdrawal.
d Wernicke's encephalopathy is rare.
e Disulfiram may be used as an adjunct to therapy.

Q113 Clinical features of stimulant abuse include:

a Convulsions.
b Myocardial infarction.
c Hypotension.
d Chronic psychosis.
e Hyperpyrexia.

Q114 Regarding carbon monoxide poisoning:

a Severity of poisoning is related to carboxyhaemoglobin level.
b To be effective hyperbaric oxygen therapy must be commenced within 24 hours.
c 'Cherry red' lips are a common finding.
d It is characterized by metabolic acidosis.
e Cardiac failure is a contraindication to hyperbaric treatment.

Q115 Regarding cyanide poisoning:

a It is commonly associated with carbon monoxide poisoning.
b Metabolic acidosis and increased anion gap suggest the diagnosis
c Amyl nitrite works by inducing the production of methaemoglobin
d Cobalt ethylenediamine tetra-acetic acid (EDTA; Kelocyanor) is a specific cyanide antidote with few side effects.
e Treatment should be withheld until blood cyanide levels are known

Q116 Concerning laburnum poisoning:

a Fatalities are common.
b Convulsions may occur.
c Poisoned children must be admitted.
d Delayed gastric lavage is indicated.
e Drowsiness may occur.

Q117 In paraquat poisoning:

a High-flow oxygen should be given.
b 15 ml of 20% solution when ingested can be fatal.
c Activated charcoal should not be given
d Skin exposure to 20% solution is usually fatal.
e Prognosis is related to serum levels.

Q118 Naloxone:

a May be given by continuous infusion.
b Can precipitate acute opioid withdrawal in an addict.
c Has a wide therapeutic index.
d Can be given intramuscularly.
e Is effective within 2 minutes.

Q119 Flumazenil:

a Acts in 30–60 seconds.
b Lasts 6–8 hours.
c Has a maximum adult dose of 1 mg.
d Should be given as a diagnostic test to all unconscious patients.
e Causes dysrhythmias.

Multiple choice questions

Q120 An oculogyric crisis can be precipitated by:

a Metoclopramide.
b Procyclidine.
c Haloperidol.
d Prochlorperazine.
e Cimetidine.

Infectious diseases

Q121 Concerning rashes:

a A solitary 'herald patch' occurs 1–2 weeks before the rash of pityriasis rosea.
b The rash of erysipelas is usually caused by *Staphylococcus aureus*.
c An eczematous rash characteristically occurs in plaques with silver-white scaling and sharply demarcated edges.
d Koplik spots are pathognomic for measles.
e The rash of rubella classically lasts for 5 days.

Q122 Concerning rashes:

a Erysipelas characteristically has a palpable edge.
b Erythema marginatum is caused by a *Staphylococcus*.
c Varicella is vesicular.
d The rash of rubella first appears on the trunk.
e A vesicular eruption can occur with barbiturate overdose.

Q123 Malaria:

a Can be excluded by negative thick and thin films stained for parasites.
b Always presents within 3 months of infection.
c Can be excluded in a patient who has taken a complete course of antimalarial prohylaxis.
d Can be excluded as a diagnosis in patients who have not travelled abroad.
e If cerebral, treatment should only be undertaken in a specialist centre.

28

Q124 Regarding herpes zoster infection:

a The rash of shingles is not infectious.
b The incubation period for chickenpox is 12–21 days.
c The rash of shingles precedes the onset of pain.
d Acyclovir is the drug of choice in severe cases.
e Fatal pneumonitis may occur in pregnant women and those on steroids.

Q125 Regarding scabies:

a The elderly are more prone to infection than the young.
b The causative organism is an arachnid.
c The web spaces are the preferred site of infection.
d Itch improves immediately on treating.
e Monosulfiram is preferable to malathion in the young and pregnant.

Q126 The following may be responsible for pyrexia of unknown origin (PUO):

a Malaria.
b Connective tissue disease.
c Münchausen's syndrome.
e Tuberculosis (TB).
e Carcinoma of the pancreas.

Q127 Regarding human immunodeficiency virus (HIV)-positive patients:

a They should not be given tetanus toxoid.
b A diagnosis of acquired immunodeficiency virus (AIDS) can be made on blood testing alone.
c Xerosis (dry skin) is a common complaint.
d Cytomegalovirus (CMV) retinitis indicates progression to AIDS.
e They should be nursed in isolation.

Q128 With regards to the viruses that cause hepatitis:

a Hepatitis C can be spread by blood transfusion.
b Normal immunoglobulin is used for the prophylaxis of hepatitis A.
c Hepatitis B is commonly transmitted during mouth-to-mouth resuscitation.
d A handkerchief effectively lowers the risk of virus transmission in mouth-to-mouth resuscitation.
e A patient with hepatitis B who is positive for the 'e' antigen has a high risk of infectivity.

Q129 Regarding meningococcal meningitis:

a Rifampicin should be given to close contacts of victims.
b Septicaemia may precede meningitis.
c Shock should be treated with IV fluids and hydrocortisone.
d Benzylpenicillin is the drug of choice.
e Adrenocortical failure may occur.

Psychiatry

Q130 The following are more likely to commit suicide:

a Older, single males.
b Drug abusers.
c Those with mental illness.
d Sufferers of chronic illnesses.
e Doctors.

Q131 Regarding the Mental Health Act 1983:

a An A&E doctor, alone, may recommend compulsory admission under section 2.
b An A&E department is a place of safety under section 136.
c Attempted suicide is an indication for compulsory admission.
d A patient in the A&E department can be detained under section 5(2).
e An A&E nurse can detain a patient for up to 6 hours under section 5(4).

Q132 Acute psychosis can be caused by:

a Non-steroidal anti-inflammatory drugs (NSAIDS).
b Cimetidine.
c Benzodiazepines.
d Corticosteroids.
e Amphetamines.

Q133 Concerning parasuicide:

a It is an act that simulates suicide but that is characterized by a low expectation of death.
b It is commoner in women than men.
c All patients should be admitted to hospital.
d There is a 20% chance of a further suicide attempt within a year.
e The SAD PERSONS scale can be used to assess the patient.

Q134 When assessing a violent patient:

a A cup of tea should be offered.
b Physical assistance should be nearby.
c An open avenue of exit should be maintained.
d Always look the patient in the eye.
e Four people are needed for forcible restraint.

Q135 The following factors favour an organic rather than a functional cause of acute psychosis:

a Disorientation.
b Vital signs normal.
c Social immodesty.
d Confabulation.
e Auditory hallucinations.

Surgery

Q136 Regarding the plain erect abdominal film:

a 10% of gallstones are visible on X-rays.
b Obliteration of the psoas shadow may indicate free fluid.
c Obstruction may be indicated by dilated loops of small bowel.
d Subdiaphragmatic free gas indicates visceral perforation.
e The spleen may be seen.

Multiple choice questions

Q137 In pancreatitis:

a Early laparotomy is indicated in severe cases.
b Parenteral pethidine is the analgesic of choice.
c Low serum calcium indicates a poor prognosis.
d Jaundice may be a presenting feature.
e Alcohol is the commonest cause in the UK.

Q138 Clinical features of testicular torsion include:

a Pyrexia.
b Vomiting as a presenting feature.
c Scrotal inflammation.
d Peak incidence between 10 and 25 years of age.
e Suprapubic pain.

Q139 In renal colic:

a Treatment with NSAIDs is appropriate.
b Haematuria is inevitable.
c The stone is visible on plain abdominal X-ray in 40% of cases.
d Vomiting can occur.
e IV antibiotics are indicated.

Q140 Small-bowel obstruction:

a Is most commonly caused by postoperative adhesions.
b Can be excluded if vomiting and abdominal distension are not present.
c Can occur as a complication of an obturator hernia.
d Can occur as a complication of a femoral hernia.
e Should be treated with a nasogastric tube.

Q141 Pyloric stenosis in children:

a Presents as projectile vomiting at birth.
b Is characterized by bile stained vomitus.
c Is commoner in girls than boys.
d Can be diagnosed by ultrasound.
e Must be treated immediately with emergency surgery.

Q142 Intussusception in children:

a Is more common in Negroes than Caucasians.
b Commonly occurs in the under-2 age group.
c Can be diagnosed on plain abdominal films.
d May be reduced by barium enema.
e Is characterized by the presence of an abdominal mass.

Paediatrics

Q143 The anterior fontanelle:

a Closes at around 10–14 months.
b Is a sensitive indicator of fluid status.
c May feel normal in critical head injury.
d If bulging, usually indicates significant intercranial pathology.
e May be tapped to relieve raised intracranial pressure.

Q144 In acute epiglottitis:

a The patient should be cannulated and receive IV ampicillin immediately.
b The causative organism is *Haemophilus influenzae*.
c The diagnosis is made in A&E by direct laryngoscopy.
d High fever and drooling of saliva are characteristic.
e Preceding coryza is common.

Q145 Regarding gastroenteritis:

a Broad-spectrum antibiotics should be prescribed if salmonella is suspected.
b Egg products are a frequent source of salmonella food poisoning.
c *Staphylococcus aureus* food poisoning results in a watery diarrhoea.
d Babies can be safely discharged if they are not vomiting.
e Diphenoxylate (Lomotil) should be prescribed routinely.

Multiple choice questions

Q146 The following suggest non-accidental injury in children:

a Epiphyseal separation of the long bones.
b Pretibial bruising.
c Subdural haematomas.
d Retinal haemorrhages.
e Fractured clavicle.

Q147 Regarding meningitis in children:

a Lumbar puncture should be performed prior to giving antibiotics.
b Neck stiffness is an unreliable sign in babies.
c The fontanelle is usually sunken.
d Papilloedema is an early sign.
e *Haemophilus* meningitis has a more rapid onset than meningococcal meninigitis.

Q148 Febrile convulsions:

a Can be excluded if the child is apyrexial.
b Only occur in the under-5 age group.
c Are associated with the development of epilepsy in 3% of cases.
d May be associated with a focal fit.
e May occur in children under 3 months of age.

Q149 The following suggest the possibility of non-accidental injury:

a Late presentation.
b Attending A&E with an adult who is not the parent.
c Torn frenulum of the upper lip.
d Labial laceration.
e Metaphyseal fractures.

Q150 Regarding urinary tract infection in children:

a Trimethoprim is the drug of choice.
b It is associated with renal tract anomalies in 40% of cases.
c All should be referred for follow up on first presentation.
d It is characterized by dysuria.
e It can predispose to scarring in the under-4 age group.

Q151 The following characterize epiglottitis rather than croup:

a Rapid onset (hours).
b Preceding coryza.
c Loud stridor.
d Muffled voice.
e Fever >38.5°C.

Q152 Regarding croup (laryngotracheobronchitis):

a Hospital admission is mandatory.
b It is commonly viral in origin.
c A 'barking' cough is characteristic.
d Pyrexia is invariable.
e Dysphagia is common.

Q153 Concerning child sexual abuse:

a Reflex anal dilatation is pathognomonic.
b It may be suggested by palatal petechiae.
c It is more common in boys.
d Approximately half the cases involve a parent or guardian.
e The diagnosis should be made in the A&E department.

Q154 Concerning childhood asthma:

a Acute exacerbation is the commonest reason for a child to be admitted to hospital in the UK.
b Peak flow rates should be measured in children above the age of 5.
c A chest X-ray must be taken in all cases when a child is to be admitted.
d Steroids should be given parenterally.
e IV fluids should be restricted to two-thirds of normal intake in severe cases.

Q155 Regarding dehydration in children:

a A 22 kg child's basic fluid requirement is 1270 ml/day.
b Urine output is a good indicator of state of hydration.
c Fluid loss in a dehydrated child should be replaced with normal saline.
d Drowsiness is an early sign.
e A shocked child should have an initial fluid bolus of 20 ml/kg given before reassessment.

Q156 Concerning bronchiolitis:

a It is the most common serious respiratory infection of children.
b Most cases occur in the spring.
c Bronchodilators should be given.
d Respiratory syncyitial virus is the most common causative organism.
e It usually affects infants in their second year.

Gynaecology

Q157 Ruptured ectopic pregnacy:

a Is characterized by profuse vaginal bleeding.
b Requires biochemical confirmation.
c Should be diagnosed by abdominal ultrasound scan.
d Requires anti-Rhesus immunization.
e Requires immediate volume replacement.

Q158 The morning-after pill:

a Frequently causes vomiting as a side-effect.
b Is effective only if taken within 24 hours of intercourse.
c Should not be administered to a patient whose menstrual period is overdue.
d Is contraindicated in those with a history of thrombotic disorder.
e May be ineffective if the patient is taking ampicillin.

Q159 Pain in the third trimester of pregnancy:

a Occurs with abruptio placentae.
b May be secondary to pre-eclampsia.
c Is common with placenta praevia.
d Due to acute appendicitis may arise in the right upper quadrant.
e Can signify premature labour.

Q160 Ectopic pregnancy:

a Can be excluded by a negative home pregnancy test.
b Is more common in users of the intrauterine device.
c Is more common following pelvic inflammatory disease.
d Is best diagnosed on vaginal ultrasound.
e Can be palpated bimanually.

Q161 Regarding pre-eclampsia:

a It may present as headaches.
b It may occur in the first 20 weeks of pregnancy.
c Disseminated intravascular coagulation (DIC) may occur.
d Proteinuria is an early sign.
e The presence of oedema is essential to making the diagnosis.

Q162 Prolapsed cord:

a May lead to fetal asphyxia.
b Requires urgent caesarean section.
c May be initially treated by instilling 500 ml saline into the bladder.
d May be treated by displacing the presenting part up into the uterus.
e May be treated by holding the cord above the presenting part.

Q163 Antepartum haemorrhage (APH):

a Is defined as bleeding >28 weeks' gestation.
b Should be assessed by vaginal examination.
c May be caused by placental abruption.
d May be complicated by DIC.
e May require anti-D immunoglobulin.

Q164 Postpartum haemorrhage (PPH):

a May be primary or secondary depending on the time since delivery.
b Is a contraindication to the administration of ergotamine.
c Routinely requires the administration of IV antibiotics.
d May require the administration of oxytocin.
e May be controlled by bimanual uterine compression.

Q165 Pelvic inflammatory disease:

a May require laparoscopy to make the diagnosis.
b Should be treated in the A&E department.
c May predispose to ectopic pregnancy.
d Is rarely acquired through sexual contact.
e May lead to infertility.

Ear, nose and throat

Q166 Regarding epistaxis:

a Control may be achieved by pressure on the bridge of the nose.
b Approximately 90% arise from Little's area.
c A full blood count should be routinely checked in the A&E department.
d A nasal pack, if inserted, should be left in place for a minimum of 48 hours.
e It is generally of no significance after nasal trauma.

Q167 Concerning quinsy:

a The anterior pillar of the fauces is obliterated.
b Dysphagia is common.
c Drainage under local anaesthetic is the treatment of choice.
d Abscess formation is usually bilateral.
e It is more common in females than males.

Q168 A subperichondrial haematoma of the ear:

a Is common in boxers.
b If seen acutely should be aspirated.
c Is otherwise known as a cauliflower ear.
d If seen after 2 days should be left to resolve.
e May lead to deafness.

Q169 Regarding swallowed foreign bodies:

a Objects traversing the pylorus are usually spontaneously expelled.
b A Foley catheter may be used to remove objects in the oesophagus.
c Mercury button batteries may be safely left in the stomach for up to 72 hours.
d Drooling is a feature of foreign bodies lodged in the oesophagus.
e X-ray examination excludes a foreign body.

Q170 Regarding Bell's palsy:

a It is usually viral in origin.
b It responds to oral steroids.
c The trigeminal nerve may be involved.
d Scalp hyperaesthesia is a feature.
e Resolution within 2 weeks is usual.

Opthalmology

Q171 A unilateral dilated pupil:

a Can occur in Holmes–Adie syndrome.
b May indicate a third nerve palsy.
c May indicate an ipsilateral Horner's syndrome.
d May occur in myasthenia gravis.
e May be a normal finding in up to 20% of the population.

Q172 Concerning the pupil:

a Organophosphate poisoning causes pupillary dilatation.
b A unilateral dilated pupil may follow an epileptic fit.
c Small pupils are more common in the elderly.
d Dilated pupils may occur following intravenous adrenaline.
e A unilateral fixed dilated pupil may follow blunt non-penetrating trauma.

Q173 In treating metallic corneal foreign bodies:

a Following local anaesthetic application a patch must be applied.
b Residual rust staining requires no treatment.
c Fluorescein staining is required to demonstrate corneal abrasions.
d Orbital X-ray is required.
e Amethocaine is a suitable local anaesthetic.

Multiple choice questions

Q174 The patient with suspected central penetrating wound to the eye:

a Should have tetanus prophylaxis.
b Should be nursed prone.
c Should receive topical anaesthetic.
d Should have intraocular pressure tested manually.
e May have a fixed dilated pupil.

Q175 Emergency treatment of chemical injury to the eye includes:

a Assessment of visual acuity.
b Urgent ophthalmic assessment of alkali burns.
c Prolonged lavage with alkali to neutralize acid contamination.
d Staining with fluorescein.
e Regular application of topical anaesthetics.

Q176 Concerning topical drugs and the eye:

a Atropine produces pupillary dilatation for 2–4 hours.
b Rose Bengal stains damaged epithelium.
c Phenylephrine causes pupillary constriction.
d Topical acyclovir is the treatment of choice for dendritic ulcer.
e Steroid drops should be prescribed for the acute red eye in the A&E department.

Q177 A sudden deterioration in visual acuity is usual with:

a Acute glaucoma.
b Bacterial conjunctivitis.
c Episcleritis.
d Cataract.
e Subconjunctival haemorrhage.

Q178 Arc eye:

a Is usually unilateral.
b Should be treated with regular mild topical anaesthetics.
c Causes short-term visual impairment.
d Is less painful after pupillary dilatation.
e Can produce abnormalities on fluorescein staining.

Q179 Orbital cellulitis:

a Is characterized by ophthalmoplegia.
b May cause cavernous sinus thrombosis.
c Responds rapidly to oral antibiotics.
e Is most commonly caused by *Staphylococcus aureus*.
e May affect branches of the trigeminal nerve.

Q180 Retinal detachment:

a Is more common in myopic eyes.
b May be secondary to intraocular melanoma.
c Results in painful loss of vision.
d May be preceded by a sensation of flashing lights.
e Can be diagnosed on fundoscopy.

Q181 Acute glaucoma:

a Is commoner in middle or later life.
b May be preceded by blurred vision or halo lights.
c Is characterized by a painless loss of vision.
d May be treated prior to transfer by pilocarpine drops 2–4% hourly.
e Responds to acetazolamide 500 mg stat.

Q182 Acute iritis (anterior uveitis):

a Is characterized by a negative Talbot's test.
b Is associated with hypopyon (pus in the anterior chamber).
c Should be treated in the A&E department with 0.5% prednisolone drops 2-hourly.
d Is characterized by a dilated, regular pupil.
e Rarely recurs.

Miscellaneous

Q183 Concerning foreign bodies:

a Olive oil instilled into the external auditory canal aids removal of insects.
b An asymptomatic child who has swallowed a coin does not require an X-ray.
c Ultrasound can be used to detect subcutaneous foreign bodies.
d Button batteries can safely be left to transit the gastrointestinal tract.
e In the tracheobronchial tree they are usually spontaneously expelled.

Q184 Concerning near drowning:

a Alcohol is a common aetiological factor.
b Hypothermia is common.
c It is associated with cervical spine injury.
d Cerebral oedema is a common complication.
e Haemolysis does not occur in seawater drownings.

Q185 Concerning diving related illnesses:

a Symptoms of the 'bends' are always evident within 2 hours of surfacing.
b Patients suspected of having air embolism should be nursed on their left side.
c The 'bends' are due to oxygen coming out of solution into the tissues.
d Air travel should be avoided for 12 hours after a dive.
e The 'bends' may cause chest pain.

Q186 Pulse oximetry:

a Can be used to indicate carboxyhaemoglobin level in the blood.
b Can be used to titrate inspired oxygen levels in patients with chronic obstructive airways disease.
c Is accurate in the presence of nail varnish.
d Predicts hypoxia when the Sp_{O_2} is less than 90%.
e Can detect low haemoglobin levels.

Q187 Immediate treatment of anaphylactic shock includes:

a IV hydrocortisone 200 mg.
b Adrenaline.
c Fluid challenges with colloid.
d Administration of high flow oxygen.
e IV aminophylline 250 mg.

Q188 Diving related illness:

a Decompression sickness is due to dissolved tissue oxygen becoming supersaturated and bubbling out of solution.
b Nitrogen narcosis may occur in the A&E department.
c Symptoms of arterial gas embolism occur within 10 minutes of ascent.
d Treatment of decompression sickness and arterial gas embolism should involve recompression.
e Otitis externa is a common illness in professional divers.

Q189 Concerning near drowning:

a It is defined as survival for at least 24 hours following a submersion event.
b 80% of drowning and near-drowning victims are male.
c Prophylactic antibiotics should be given.
d Treatment will depend on whether the patient was immersed in salt or fresh water.
e 'Wet drowning' indicates that the whole body was immersed.

Q190 Major burns:

a First aid includes cooling the affected area under running cold water for 10 minutes.
b Fluid loss is related to body weight.
c IM NSAIDs should be used for analgesia.
d Escharotomy should be performed through all full-thickness burns.
e Prophylactic parenteral antibiotics should be given.

Multiple choice questions

Q191 In electric shock:

a Alternating current is more likely to produce ventricular fibrillation than direct current.
b Cardiac arrest from lightning strike is due to ventricular fibrillation.
c Direct current produces a large entry and small exit wound.
d Renal failure may be a complication.
e Bone injury should be excluded.

Q192 Hydrofluoric acid burns:

a Are non-painful.
b Most commonly occur on the upper limbs.
c May be associated with systemic toxicity.
d Should be treated with copious lavage.
e May be treated with calcium gluconate gel.

Q193 Concerning lignocaine for local anaesthesia:

a 10 ml of 1% solution contains 10 mg lignocaine.
b The maximum safe recommended dose is 10 mg/kg.
c Overdosage may result in convulsions.
d Higher doses may be used if mixed with adrenaline.
e It causes methaemoglobinaemia.

Q194 Regarding tetanus:

a In the UK schoolchildren should have a tetanus booster before leaving school.
b A man who has completed a full course of tetanus immunization 7 years ago and who now has a small wound on his finger does not require any further immunization.
c Antitetanus immunoglobulin should be given to the non-immunized patient who has suffered a clean wound.
d A patient who is allergic to tetanus toxoid should not be given antitetanus immunoglobulin.
e Removing of devitalized tissue from a deep wound is of prime importance in preventing tetanus.

Q195 The following dressings are appropriate:

a Clingfilm for an extensive burn.
b Paraffin gauze for a minor burn.
c Liquid parafin for a facial burn.
d Paraffin gauze for an incised facial wound that has been sutured.
e Application of silver sulphadiazine cream and a plastic bag for a hand burn.

Q196 Entonox:

a Is contraindicated in pneumothorax.
b Is administered by a patient-demand valve.
c Is contraindicated in Caisson's disease.
d Should be shaken before use in cold weather.
e Causes significant hypotension.

Q197 Dog bites on the hand:

a Require tetanus prophylaxis.
b Do not require antibiotic therapy.
c Require primary closure.
d Should be X-rayed.
e May result in osteomyelitis.

Q198 Regarding burns:

a Burns to hands should be immobilized in a splint.
b Blisters should always be deroofed and aspirated.
c Paraffin gauze is a suitable dressing for partial thickness burns to the forearm.
d Full-thickness burns look like leather.
e Burns to the face should be dressed with silver sulphadiazine cream.

Q199 Torticollis may be:

a Congenital.
b Secondary to cervical disc prolapse.
c Posttraumatic.
d Associated with eye disease.
e Associated with upper-limb paraesthesiae.

Multiple choice questions

Q200 Concerning needlestick injury:

a Injury caused by a hollow needle is of more concern than that caused by a solid needle.
b If hepatitis status of the victim is unknown then immunoglobulin should be given.
c Tetanus prophylaxis should be given.
d Seroconversion to HIV-positive status occurs in 0.1% of cases.
e Early local incision of the wound is required.

MULTIPLE CHOICE ANSWERS

Trauma and Orthopaedics

General

Q1
a T **b** T **c** T **d** T **e** F

The Salter-Harris classification relates to epiphyseal plate injuries (Fig. 1). In general, increasing grade relates to increasing severity of injury. All are evident on X-ray except type V. Growth arrest with subsequent limb deformity is a recognized complication. Slipped upper femoral epiphysis is a type I injury. Type II injuries are the most common. By the age of 22 years the epiphyses are closed and therefore by definition a Salter-Harris fracture cannot happen.

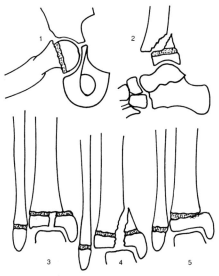

Fig. 1 Salter-Harris classification of epiphyseal plate injuries. Type 1: The whole epiphysis is separated from the shaft. Type 2: The epiphysis is displaced, carrying with it a small, triangular metaphyseal fragment (the commonest injury). Type 3: Separation of part of the epiphysis. Type 4: Separation of part of the epiphysis, with a metaphyseal fragment. Type 5: Crushing of part of the epiphysis.

Q2
a T b T c T d F e T

Sudeck's atrophy is due to an abnormal sympathetic response to trauma It is characterized by a warm, pink glazed extremity, which is tender with a restricted range of movement. It most commonly complicates Colles fracture but can occur secondary to any extremity fracture. It is a self-limiting condition, usually resolving within 12 months. Physiotherapy should be used to minimize permanent restriction of movement. Severe cases may show some response to guanethidine block.

Q3
a T b T c T d F e T

Compartment syndrome is caused by occlusion to venous and later arterial blood flow within a closed tissue space (e.g. the forearm, which is enveloped within an indistensible deep fascia). The early signs are pain and paraesthesia. Muscle swelling and necrosis lead to ischaemic contracture. The condition is commonly described in the forearm (Volkmann's ischaemic contracture of the forearm flexors), but may also occur in the leg. It commonly follows long bone fracture. Loss of distal pulses is a late sequela and cannot therefore be used to diagnose the condition. Tissue pressure may be measured directly to confirm the diagnosis, but is not essential to the management.

Q4
a T b F c T d T e T

Q5
a F b F c F d F e F

The patient with rib fractures requires a chest X-ray if physical examination suggests pneumothorax or multiple fractures, if surgical emphysema is present or if the mechanism and force of injury give cause for concern. X-ray is rarely required in the young with blunt chest trauma due to sport but should be carried out more readily in the frail elderly. Intercostal block may be dramatically effective in relieving the pain of rib fractures. Strapping of the chest can relieve pain but does not improve outcome and may increase the chance of pulmonary complications. Although lung infection may follow rib fractures, prophylactic antibiotics are not indicated.

Q6
a F b F c T d F e T

Jagged lacerations over the metacarpophalangeal joints caused by punching someone in the teeth are the commonest cause of septic arthritis in the hand. Tendon sheath infections characteristically cause excruciating pain on passive extension of the fingers. A paronychia is a superficial infection over the lateral nailfold. The usual causative organism is *Staphylococcus aureus*. β-Haemolytic streptococci, anaerobes and *Candida albicans* are other causes. Early paronychia can be treated with elevation and antibiotics but as soon as an abscess has formed it should be drained. Herpetic whitlows are caused by a herpes simplex infection of the fingers.

Q7
a T b F c F d F e T

The haematoma block is a simple technique in which local anaesthetic is injected between the fragments of fractured bone. A venous tourniquet should not be used. Osteomyelitis has not been reported using this technique. However, risk of disseminating infection precludes the use of this block if the fracture is compound. When used for a Colles fracture, the fracture should be approached from the dorsal aspect to avoid damage to the more complex volar structures. The haematoma block can also be used in other sites, such as the metacarpals or the phalanges.

Q8
a F b F c T d F e F

Bier's blockade is a safe procedure if performed correctly. Several fatalities occurred in the 1980s when bupivacaine was being used. It is now recommended that the local anaesthetic used should be prilocaine, a less cardiotoxic drug. The first sign of local anaesthetic toxicity is usually perioral tingling followed by fitting. A cannula should be placed in both arms, one through which to give the anaesthetic and one as a route for any emergency drugs. Two doctors should be present throughout the procedure, the first to give the anaesthetic and the second to perform the reduction or operation. The cuff should be inflated to a pressure of 100 mmHg above the systolic pressure and should not be deflated until at least 20 minutes after the local anaesthetic injection.

Q9
a F **b** T **c** F **d** F **e** F

The Revised Trauma Score is the sum of weighted values for Glasgow Coma Score, systolic blood pressure and respiratory rate. The range is 0 (dead) to 7.84 (normal). Many victims of major trauma have an initially normal value before decompensation occurs. The initial value is used in the Major Trauma Outcome Study.

Q10
a F **b** T **c** F **d** T **e** F

The Glasgow Coma Score uses assessment of verbal, motor and eye response to stimuli, to give a total score ranging from 3 (no response to any stimulus) to 15 (normal response to all stimuli). A score of less than 8 indicates coma. There are four possible eye responses, five possible verbal responses and six possible motor responses. An eye response of 3 indicates eye opening to speech.

Q11
a F **b** F **c** T **d** F **e** F

Greenstick fractures are incomplete angulated fractures of long bones. They occur in the soft resilient bones of children. A torus fracture occurs when the cortex of a bone buckles but does not fracture. This produces a small bump or torus on X-ray.

The upper limb

Q12
a T **b** F **c** F **d** F **e** F

Shoulder injuries require early mobilization to prevent the complication of frozen shoulder, characterized by stiffness and marked restriction in the range of movement. Once established, frozen shoulder may take up to 18 months to resolve. Most acromioclavicular subluxations and dislocations are treated conservatively. Fractured clavicle is initially treated in a broad arm sling, although a figure-of-eight bandage may be applied in an attempt to improve the position of the fracture. Complete rotator cuff tears are best repaired, although the diagnosis is often made late. Painful arc syndrome is characterized by pain on abduction between 45 and 160°.

Q13
a T **b** F **c** T **d** F **e** F

Posterior dislocation is rare in comparison to anterior dislocation. It is classically described as a complication of an epileptic fit or electrocution. It is not always evident on the standard anteroposterior view, the humeral head appearing rotated (the 'light bulb' sign). The Bankhart lesion (tearing of the capsule away from its attachment to the glenoid) is associated with anterior dislocation. Reduction can be achieved with sedation and analgesia. General anaesthesia is rarely required. The integrity of the axillary nerve must be tested before and after reduction. Abduction of the shoulder is usually too painful, therefore paraesthesia over the insertion of the deltoid is tested, not over the tip of the shoulder.

Q14
a T **b** T **c** F **d** T **e** T

The ulnar nerve is most vulnerable at the elbow and may be injured with a fracture or a dislocation. The ulnar nerve supplies the hypothenar muscles, the interossei, the medial two lumbricals and adductor pollicis in the hand. The median nerve supplies all of the other thenar muscles and the lateral two lumbricals. Radial nerve injury may cause wrist drop and weak extension of the fingers.

Q15
a F **b** T **c** T **d** T **e** F

Early mobilization of an elbow haemarthrosis may lead to myositis ossificans.

Q16
a T **b** T **c** T **d** F **e** T

Radial head fracture is usually caused by a fall on to the outstretched hand. Pain is worse on pronation and supination and when direct pressure is applied over the radial head. The fracture is often missed, especially when undisplaced. Coned views may be required to make the diagnosis. The joint may be aspirated to relieve pain and aid mobilization. Five to 10° of extensor lag is common after the injury and full recovery may not occur.

Multiple choice answers

Q17
a F **b** T **c** F **d** T **e** F

Pulled elbow is a clinical diagnosis. There is no recognized radiological appearance. Undisplaced fracture of the olecranon is treated in an above elbow plaster. Posterior dislocation of the elbow may be complicated by median or ulnar nerve palsy.

Q18
a F **b** T **c** F **d** T **e** T

A Monteggia fracture–dislocation involves fracture of the proximal ulna with an associated dislocation of the radial head. It is usually caused by a fall on to the outstretched hand. Missed fractures may be associated with subsequent development of an ulnar nerve palsy. A Galeazzi fracture–dislocation involves fracture of the distal radius with an associated dislocation of the distal ulnar. Both fractures require internal fixation and both may be complicated by compartment syndrome.

Q19
a T **b** T **c** T **d** F **e** T

A Colles fracture is a break in the distal radius within 3 cm of the wrist, more common in elderly women. It is characterized by impaction and dorsal and radial displacement of the distal fragment. Indications for reduction include radial shortening and 10° or more of dorsal tilt of the joint line. The age, degree of mobility and general condition of the patient should always be taken into consideration when assessing the need for manipulation. Reduction is achieved using local, regional or general anaesthesia, the wrist being immobilized in pronation, ulnar deviation and slight flexion. Complications include malunion, delayed rupture of extensor pollicis longus, Sudeck's atrophy, carpal tunnel syndrome and persistent stiffness of the shoulder, elbow and wrist.

Q20
a T **b** F **c** T **d** F **e** T

Barton's fracture is a fracture of the distal radius involving the articular surface. The dorsal portion of the articular surface of the radius is displaced and internal fixation is often required. Smith described a fracture of the distal radius in which the distal portion of the bone is displaced in a volar direction: it is treated by closed reduction initially with the wrist in extension in an above-elbow plaster.

Q21
a F **b** F **c** F **d** F **e** F

Scaphoid fracture results from a fall on to the outstretched hand, or from a 'kick-back' injury. Tenderness in the anatomical snuffbox is common after wrist injury but only a few patients with this sign have a scaphoid fracture. Fifty per cent of fractures occur through the waist (38% occur in the proximal half and 12% in the distal half). Fractures of the waist and proximal pole may result in avascular necrosis of the proximal section in patients with a distal blood supply.

Q22
a T **b** T **c** T **d** F **e** T

De Quervain's tenosynovitis affects the tendons of extensor pollicis brevis and abductor pollicis longus. It produces a positive Finkelstein's test (pain on opposed extension and abduction of the thumb). The condition is most common in those who repetitively use their wrists and thumbs, such as keyboard operators. It may respond to rest and NSAIDs, steroid injection or immobilization in a scaphoid plaster for 14 days.

Q23
a T **b** T **c** T **d** T **e** T

Carpal dislocations are uncommon. They usually result from a
high-speed fall on to the outstretched hand. Two main types are
recognized. The first is characterized by dorsal dislocation of the
metacarpals, the distal row of the carpus and part of the proximal
row. The term 'peri' is used in this group to describe structures in the
proximal row which are undisplaced. One of the carpal bones may
fracture, part of it remaining in alignment and part dislocating. The
second group is characterized by the realignment of the distal row
with the radius and a consequent dislocation of the proximal row
(e.g. dislocation of the lunate, scaphoid or both, or dislocation of the
lunate and part of the scaphoid). Dislocation of the lunate is the
commonest type and is sometimes missed due to failure to interpret
the lateral wrist view correctly. Median nerve involvement is
common.

Q24
a T **b** F **c** T **d** F **e** T

Carpal tunnel syndrome is caused by compression of the median
nerve as it passes beneath the flexor retinaculum at the wrist. It
commonly causes pain and paraesthesia at night and is associated
with pregnancy. Locally injected steroids can bring some relief, but
carpal tunnel release may be necessary. Wrist drop is due to radial
nerve palsy.

Q25
a T **b** F **c** F **d** T **e** F

The ulnar collateral ligament is frequently injured in skiing accidents
when the thumb is forcibly abducted by the strap of the ski pole. The
ligament stabilizes the thumb. A tear results in a weak pinch grip.
Complete tears should be surgically repaired at formal operation.
Partial tears can be treated in a plaster thumb spica.

Q26
a F **b** T **c** T **d** F **e** F

Bennett's fracture results from an abduction injury to the thumb. It involves the trapezometacarpal joint with proximal and lateral subluxation of the thumb metacarpal. It can be treated by closed manipulation with the thumb maintained in abduction in a Bennett's plaster. Open or percutaneous fixation is often required if a good position cannot be maintained.

Q27
a F **b** F **c** F **d** F **e** F

Flexor tendon injuries should be repaired under full aseptic technique and tourniquet by an experienced surgeon. The distal interphalangeal joint (DIPJ) is flexed by flexor digitorum profundus (FDP) the proximal interphalangeal joint (PIPJ) is flexed by FDP and flexor digitorum superficialis (FDS). Mallet deformity results from division of the extensor tendon at or about the DIPJ. A fracture with displacement of the insertion of the extensor tendon will result in the same deformity. Extension at the metacarpophalangeal joint is produced by the intrinsic muscles of the hand as well as the extensors. To overcome this intrinsic extension the hand should be placed palm down on a flat surface whilst testing extension. Boutonnière deformity is due to a ruptured central slip of the extensor mechanism and should be repaired early for best results. The hand should always be immobilized in the position of function with the metacarpophalangeal joints flexed to 90° and the IPJs extended to 180°.

Q28
a F **b** F **c** T **d** T **e** F

The most important principle in the management of minor finger injuries is early mobilization. Some support is also necessary. This can be accomplished using buddy strapping (the finger is taped to its neighbour), or by using a Bedford splint (a tube of tubigrip stitched along its length to divide it into two lengthways). PIPJ injuries tend to lead to more disability because of the large range of movement at this joint. A mallet splint should be worn initially for 6 weeks.

Multiple choice answers

Pelvis and lower limb

Q29
a F b T c F d T e T

There are three types of major pelvic fracture – the 'butterfly fracture', resulting from direct anteroposterior compression, 'bucket-handle' fractures of the hemipelvices and vertical shearing injuries. These last have the highest mortality. Initial clinical examination including springing the pelvis may not indicate an underlying fracture, hence the need for a pelvic X-ray as part of the primary survey. Pelvic fractures are associated with injuries to the urogenital system, the small bowel, rectum and diaphragm. Massive haemorrhage is also frequently seen.

Q30
a F b T c F d T e T

Posterior dislocation of the hip characteristically produces flexion, adduction and internal rotation of the leg. It is 10–20 times more common than anterior dislocation and usually results from forces transmitted up the line of the femur. Associated injuries include fracture of the patella, posterior acetabular lip and femoral shaft. Sciatic nerve damage may also occur, resulting in decreased sensation below the knee and loss of dorsiflexion of the foot. Reduction is usually carried out under general anaesthetic, although an attempt at reduction under intravenous sedation and analgesia may be warranted if a delay is anticipated in arranging a general anaesthetic. After reduction the patient should be admitted for rest and light skin traction.

Q31
a F b F c F d T e T

Perthes disease is avascular necrosis of the femoral head. It is four
times more common in boys than girls and usually presents between
the age of 4 and 8 with a limp, hip pain and reduced hip movements.
The earliest radiographic changes are increased epiphyseal density
and widening of the joint space. Treatment is usually conservative
using traction.

Slipped upper femoral epiphysis occurs in an older age group
between the age of 10 and 18. It is slightly more common in boys
than girls and is more common in excessively tall or very fat children
with delayed gonadal development. The child usually presents with
hip, groin or knee pain together with a limp. On examination the
affected leg appears externally rotated and short, and abduction and
internal rotation of the hip are limited. Treatment is surgical by
internal fixation with or without osteotomy.

Q32
a F b T c T d F e T

Fractured neck of femur usually presents with shortening and external
rotation of the leg. Intracapsular fractures which disrupt the main
arterial supply may result in avascular necrosis. An impacted fracture
may present with persisting pain several weeks after the initial injury.
Bruising over the greater trochanter is a late sign and only occurs in
extracapsular fractures.

Q33
a T b F c T d T e T

The force required to fracture the femoral shaft is considerable and
may have also caused a pelvic fracture. A fracture that is not open is
usually associated with 0.5–1 litre of blood loss. Considerable pain
relief and effective immobilization can be achieved by the use of a
traction splint. Fat embolism is common in femoral shaft fractures
and should be suspected if the patient has a hypoxic episode.
Underlying pathology should always be considered with femoral shaft
fractures in the over-50 age group.

Multiple choice answers

Q34
a F **b** T **c** F **d** F **e** T

The medial collateral ligament is the most frequently damaged ligament in the knee. Valgus forces can produce a widespread injury to the medial collateral and anterior cruciate ligaments and to the medial meniscus. McMurray's test may be used to diagnose a meniscal injury. However, tenderness over the joint line may be more sensitive in the acutely swollen knee. A tense knee swelling immediately after an injury suggests haemarthrosis. Aspiration under strict aseptic conditions may help in diagnosing a fracture if fat globules are seen in the blood, as well as giving the patient symptomatic relief.

Q35
a T **b** T **c** T **d** T **e** T

The knee is a frequent source of complaint in the adolescent age group. Osgood–Schlatter disease is a traction apophysitis of the site of insertion of the patella tendon. Resolution usually occurs following temporary restriction of exercise. Chondromalacia patellae is another cause of knee pain in the adolescent. The articular cartilage of the patella is softer than normal, resulting in pain and crepitus in the anterior knee. Hip conditions should never be overlooked when examining the child as pain is often referred to the knee. Henoch–Schönlein purpura can cause a flitting arthritis affecting the large joints.

Q36
a T **b** T **c** T **d** F **e** T

Open tibial fractures are common as so much of the bone runs subcutaneously. The proximity of the popliteal artery to the upper tibia means it is susceptible to damage with upper tibial fractures. Ischaemia of the distal fragment is a rare complication of tibial fracture. Undisplaced fractures in children are usually treated in a long leg cast which can be converted into a walking plaster as soon as there is evidence of callus on the radiographs. Stress fractures occur most commonly in the metatarsal shafts, the distal tibia and the femoral neck.

Q37
a T **b** F **c** T **d** F **e** T

Achilles tendon rupture is commonest in middle-aged men following sudden muscular activity. The rupture usually occurs 4–8 cm above the site of insertion. Characteristically the patient is unable to stand on tiptoe. Sometimes, however, this movement can be achieved using extensor hallicis longus. It is therefore necessary to perform Simmonds test to exclude a diagnosis of complete rupture of the Achilles tendon: the calf is squeezed between the thumb and index finger. If the tendon is completely divided there will be no plantar flexion of the foot. Treatment can either be surgical or conservative with an above knee equinus plaster.

Q38
a F **b** T **c** F **d** F **e** F

Most ankle injuries are caused by inversion forces. A simple sprain should resolve within 10 days. A complete lateral ligament tear, however, may need surgical repair or plaster fixation for up to 6 weeks. If the ankle is dislocated then this should be reduced as soon as possible, using intravenous sedation and analgesia. Any delay significantly increases the chances of skin necrosis over the dislocation. A fracture of the fibula above the distal tibiofibular joint results in a stable ankle and should be treated conservatively. The Maisonneuve fracture complex is a fracture of the medial malleolus associated with a fracture of the neck of the fibula. It is caused by a pronation/lateral rotation injury.

Q39
a F b T c T d T e T

Fractures of the calcaneum are usually caused by a fall from a height on to the heels. The same forces can cause pelvic, hip and spinal fractures which should not be overlooked. Böhler's angle (Fig. 2; the angle between a line drawn from the anterior articular process of the calcaneus to the posterior articular surface and a line drawn between the posterior articular surface and the superior angle of the calcaneal tuberosity) is normally about 40° and is decreased in fractures which flatten the profile of the heel. Calcaneal fractures often involve the subtalar joint. The extent of this involvement is best determined using a CT scan. Secondary osteoarthritis following this injury is unfortunately very common.

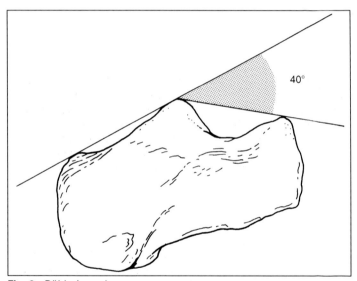

Fig. 2 Böhler's angle.

Q40
a F b F c T d F e T

Undisplaced metatarsal fractures should be treated symptomatically and may be managed in a support bandage. A March fracture usually occurs in the neck of the second or third metatarsal. Avulsion fracture of the base of the fifth metatarsal is the commonest fracture in the foot. It is caused when peroneus brevis contracts fiercely to correct inversion of the foot and so avulses its bony attachment. The Jones fracture is a fracture of the fifth metatarsal base distal to the intermetatarsal joint which occurs in athletes in training and frequently results in non-union. Fractures of the talar neck are classically associated with car accidents and plane crashes when forced dorsiflexion of the foot occurs against the pedal or rudder.

Head and spine

Q41
a F b T c T d F e F

The diagnosis of a basal skull fracture is usually clinical. Anosmia may result from tearing of the olfactory fibres as they emerge through the cribriform plate on the undersurface of the frontal lobes. Other signs include bleeding from the ear, haemotympanum, cerebrospinal fluid rhinorrhoea or otorrhoea, bruising over the mastoid (Battle's sign) and periorbital bruising ('racoon eyes'). Subconjunctival, not subhyaloid, haemorrhage may also occur.

Q42
a T b T c F d F e T

All patients with new skull fractures should be admitted for observation. The patient with a skull fracture has a 3% chance of intracranial haemorrhage if the GCS is normal but this rises to 25% if the GCS is decreased. Urgent CT scan should be performed if the patient has abnormal neurological signs or the GCS is decreased.

Q43
a F b T c T d F e T

Accepted indications for skull X-ray include loss of consciousness, amnesia, drowsiness at the time of assessment, persistent vomiting and neurological symptoms and signs. An X-ray should also be performed in those suffering from alcohol intoxication and any other patient for whom an adequate history cannot be obtained. A scalp laceration of 5 cm alone is not an indication for an X-ray. It should be borne in mind that local admitting policies and the availability of CT scanning may result in some variation from these guidelines.

Q44
a F b T c F d F e F

Although of less significance than localized seizures, any patient who has a grand mal fit following a head injury should be discussed with the neurosurgical team. Post-traumatic amnesia, skull fracture on X-ray and persistent vomiting (most common in children) are reasons for admission following a head injury.

Q45
a T b T c F d T e T

The dose of mannitol is 0.5–1.0 g/kg of a 20% solution given over 15–20 minutes. At best this may temporarily reduce cerebral oedema and may therefore be useful where surgery is likely to be delayed. Mannitol should not normally be given without discussion with the neurosurgical team. Side effects of mannitol include a paradoxical rise in intracranial pressure and systemic hypotension.

Q46
a T b F c F d F e F

'Whiplash' injuries are commonly caused by a rear shunt in a road traffic accident. Cervical spine fractures are rare with this injury. X-ray examination should be confined to those with symptoms immediately after the crash. The central cord syndrome is rare under the age of 60. The majority of patients have a full recovery within 10–14 days of injury. The mainstay of treatment is analgesia and early mobilization. Soft collars, if used at all, should only be used for 48 hours. Although commonly stated to predispose to early cervical spondylosis, there is no evidence of an association between these two common conditions.

Q47
a F **b** F **c** F **d** F **e** F

Neurogenic shock results from interruption of descending sympathetic pathways leading to loss of vasomotor tone and sympathetic input to the heart. Consequent vasodilatation of visceral and lower extremity vessels results in hypotension. Fluid infusion is not effective in restoring normal blood pressure and may indeed result in fluid overload, although vasopressors may be helpful. Priapism is a rare sign but is strongly associated with a severe spinal cord injury. Maximum neurological deficit often does not develop immediately but takes many hours. The cervical spine cannot be considered adequately immobilized in a semirigid neck collar alone. Sandbags and tape should also be used.

Q48
a T **b** T **c** F **d** F **e** T

Spinal fractures commonly occur at the junction between mobile and relatively fixed segments of the vertebral column, such as the cervicothoracic and the thoracolumbar junctions. If anterior wedging is less than 15° or the anterior vertebral height is greater than two-thirds of the posterior vertebral height, the fracture is usually stable. Jefferson's fracture is a 'blow-out' fracture of the atlas caused by direct compression. In unilateral facet dislocation the superior vertebral body is seen to overlap the one below by approximately one-third.

Q49
a F **b** T **c** F **d** F **e** F

In the resuscitation of major trauma the neck should be brought carefully into the neutral position before being immobilized. It is not possible to achieve adequate immobilization of the cervical spine in other positions and airway maintenance may also be more difficult. Type I odontoid fractures occur above the base of the odontoid and are usually stable. Type II occur at the base and are usually unstable and type III fractures extend into the vertebral body. The 'hangman's fracture' is a fracture of the pedicle of C2.

Q50
a T b F c T d T e T

Pseudosubluxation of C2 on C3 occurs in 40% of children under the age of 7 and persists in 20% of children under 16. It is also seen, less commonly, between C3 and C4. In cases where there may be a high suspicion of cervical spine trauma, either on the basis of symptoms or signs, a lateral cervical spine X-ray alone may not be sufficient to exclude significant injury. An anteroposterior and peg view should be performed as routine and CT may be needed. It has been suggested that portable cervical spine films will miss 5–10% of fractures. The 'swimmer's' view is taken through the axilla with the arm closest to the X-ray tube fully abducted. It is used to visualize the lower cervical spine if this area cannot be seen on the standard lateral film. The upper limit of normal for the distance between the anterior aspect of the odontoid and the anterior arch of C1 is 3 mm in adults.

Maxillofacial injuries

Q51
a T b T c T d T e T

Laryngeal fractures are rare and result from attempted hanging or from direct trauma to the neck such as occurs in a road traffic accident with impact of the neck on the steering wheel. Airway management may be difficult and endotracheal intubation impossible. A cricothyroidotomy may also not be possible. In this scenario an emergency tracheostomy may be required.

Q52
a T b T c T d T e T

The so called 'blow-out' fracture results from direct trauma to the eye, (often with a squash ball or shuttlecock), the transmitted pressure causing the eyeball to fracture the thin walled orbital floor. The trauma to the eye may result in a hyphaema. Herniation of the inferior oblique and inferior rectus muscles into the maxillary antrum results in double vision on upward gaze. The teardrop sign is caused by this oedematous, herniated tissue and may be seen on X-ray together with opacity of the maxillary antrum.

Q53
a F **b** F **c** T **d** T **e** F

The patient with a swollen injured nose is a common sight in the
A&E department. Bleeding from a broken nose usually stops
spontaneously. If cerebrospinal fluid is mixed with the blood, a
nasoethmoid fracture should be suspected. If a septal haematoma is
present, it should be drained. Blood in the nasal septum greatly
increases the chance of infection and septal collapse. Septal deviation
is an indication for reduction as it may cause airway obstruction.
Cosmetic deformity should be assessed after 5 days by an ear, nose
and throat specialist when much of the swelling will have reduced. A
decision regarding reduction can then be made. X-rays are not
usually required for these clinical decisions. Some parties maintain
that X-rays need to be taken for medicolegal reasons. We take a
photograph of the injury if legal action is expected.

Q54
a F **b** F **c** T **d** F **e** F

Fractures of the mandible are usually multiple and are most often
best seen with a dental panoramic view. A dislocated mandible can
be unilateral or bilateral. The patient will have an open mouth which
he or she will not be able to close.

Q55
a T **b** T **c** F **d** T **e** F

Fifty per cent of reimplanted teeth will survive. Until reimplantation
the patient should be advised either to keep the tooth between the
gum and cheek or to put it in a container of milk. The tooth can be
replaced in its socket in the A&E department and held with silver foil
before being referred to a dentist for definitive treatment. A patient
who has suffered major trauma and has a missing tooth should have
a chest X-ray to exclude aspiration of the tooth into the lungs.

Multiple choice answers

Trauma resuscitation

Q56
a F b F c F d F e F

The priorities in trauma resuscitation are airway with cervical spine control, then breathing, then circulation with haemorrhage control. Peripheral lines are preferable to central lines in terms of ease and speed of insertion, low complication rates and speed of infusion. Cervical collars should be left on until the admitting team have assessed the patient. Failure to visualize C7–T1 on standard views should prompt the taking of swimmer's views.

Q57
a T b F c F d F e F

An occlusive dressing sealed at three sides to the chest wall will act as a flutter valve and will allow air out of the chest but not in. A chest drain should be inserted on the ipsilateral side away from the wound. Surgical closure of small defects may not be necessary. A chest drain should be inserted on the contralateral side only if indicated.

Q58
a F b F c T d F e T

Tension pneumothorax is a clinical diagnosis and is identified by tracheal deviation away from the side of the pneumothorax, respiratory distress, unilateral absence of breath sounds, distended neck veins and cyanosis. Treatment should not be delayed to obtain an X-ray. The immediate treatment is insertion of a needle into the second intercostal space in the mid clavicular line, followed later by placement of a chest drain.

Q59
a F b T c F d F e T

Cardiac tamponade is often a late diagnosis. It is characterized by Beck's triad of venous pressure elevation, muffled heart sounds and decreasing arterial pressure. The initial treatment is by needle pericardiocentesis, followed later by formal thoracotomy. Removal of as little as 15–20 ml of blood may be beneficial.

Q60
a T b F c T d T e T

ECG signs of myocardial contusion include multiple ventricular premature beats, unexplained sinus tachycardia, atrial fibrillation, bundle branch block (usually right) and ST segment changes. Raised cardiac enzymes are characteristic (cardiac specific enzymes, since concomitant skeletal muscle damage causes raised muscle enzyme levels). Death may occur due to dysrhythmias.

Q61
a T b F c F d T e T

Cricothyroidotomy provides adequate oxygenation for up to 45 minutes but does not allow adequate ventilation, so Pco_2 levels increase with time.

Q62
a F b F c T d T e F

Relative contraindications to peritoneal lavage include advanced cirrhosis, bleeding diatheses, morbid obesity and previous abdominal surgery. False-positive results occur in 2–3% of cases and false negatives in 2%. The test is considered positive if the effluent fluid contains more than 100 000 red blood cells per cubic millimetre. Pelvic fracture may produce a false positive result in the absence of intraperitoneal injury. False negative results usually occur in isolated bladder or bowel injury. Signs of peritoneal irritation after major trauma are an absolute indication for laparotomy.

Q63
a T b F c F d T e F

A nasogastric tube and bladder catheter should always be inserted prior to diagnostic peritoneal lavage. A lower midline incision is used. A negative result does not exclude intra-abdominal or retroperitoneal pathology.

Multiple choice answers

Q64
a F **b** F **c** F **d** T **e** T

Genitourinary injury should be suspected in any trauma patient who
has macroscopic haematuria. However, the quantity of blood in the
urine is not usually related to the severity of the trauma. There may
be no haematuria with renal pedicle injury and renal vascular
thrombosis secondary to blunt trauma. Some 85–90% of renal
injuries can be managed conservatively. Bladder injuries most
frequently occur in road traffic accidents when the patient has a full
bladder. Damage to the male anterior urethra should be suspected
with a history of falling astride an object such as a manhole cover.
The diagnosis can be confirmed with a retrograde urethrogram.

Q65
a F **b** F **c** T **d** T **e** T

The odontoid peg usually fractures in the same plane as CT 'cuts'
and fractures may therefore be missed; for the same reason, some
skull vault fractures may only be revealed by plain skull X-rays.
Extradural haematomas present with an area of increased density
convex inwards and limited by dural adhesions to the skull. Subdural
haematomas become isodense with brain 10–20 days following injury
and hyperdense thereafter.

Q66
a T **b** F **c** T **d** T **e** T

Retroperitoneal injuries may not be evident on initial assessment. The
retroperitoneal space contains the aorta, vena cava, pancreas, kidneys,
ureters and sections of the colon and duodenum. It is not sampled by
peritoneal lavage. Radiological signs of retroperitoneal injury include
fractures of the lumbar spinous processes and obliteration of the
psoas shadows. Periumbilical bruising (Cullen's sign) and flank
bruising, (Grey Turner sign) are signs of retroperitoneal haemorrhage,
but are usually late and are unlikely to be found in the A&E
department.

Q67
a T b F c F d T e T

Urethral trauma is more common in men than women due to the longer length of the male urethra. Up to 20% of pelvic fractures may be associated with a posterior urethral injury. Frank haematuria rather than microscopic haematuria indicates a clinically significant urinary tract injury and retrograde urethrography is mandatory before any attempt at catheterization is made. Urethral injuries are rare in women but should be suspected if vaginal bleeding or laceration is found. Vaginal examination, which is mandatory, may demonstrate bony fragments from a pelvic fracture.

Medicine

General and cardiology

Q68
a F b T c T d F e F

Contraindications to thrombolysis include recent haemorrhage, trauma or surgery, bleeding disorders, cerebrovascular disease (especially recent), possible peptic ulceration, severe hypertension, cavitating pulmonary disease, acute pancreatitis, diabetic retinopathy, severe liver disease and oesophageal varices. Neither streptokinase nor anistreplase (APSAC) should be given between 5 days and 12 months following previous treatment with either drug.

Q69
a T b T c F d F e T

Myocardial infarction is now the commonest cause of death in the UK. A diagnosis may be made if two of three components – history, ECG and cardiac enzymes – are positive. Therefore, the cardiac enzymes are positive and the history appropriate, a positive ECG is not required for the diagnosis. A temperature of up to 38°C occurs due to muscle necrosis and may last up to 7 days. Creatinine kinase peaks within 24 hours, aspartate aminotransferase (AST or SGOT) peaks at 24–48 hours and lactate dehydrogenase peaks at 3–4 days, remaining elevated for 10–14 days. Complete heart block is associated with inferior myocardial infarction.

Multiple choice answers

Q70
a T b F c F d T e F

Cardiogenic shock is usually associated with extensive and irreversible myocardial damage. It is more common after an anterior infarct. The tissue hypoxia results in a metabolic acidosis. Treatment is usually with sympathomimetics such as dopamine and dobutamine but the prognosis is poor.

Q71
a T b T c F d F e T

Adrenocortical failure may develop insidiously, only manifesting itself when a crisis intervenes, often precipitated by infection, trauma or surgery. The commonest cause in the UK is autoimmune Addison's disease. Treatment is with hydrocortisone combined with fludrocortisone (which has a mineralocorticoid action). In a crisis IV normal saline is required in addition to steroids.

Q72
a T b F c T d T e T

Although 50 ml of a 50% solution is the standard treatment for adult hypoglycaemic coma, hypertonic glucose solutions may precipitate cerebral oedema, especially in children. Because of the rapid response to glucose the dose may be titrated to give the desired effect whilst avoiding a rebound hyperglycaemia. A serum glucose in the normal range does not exclude hypoglycaemia. In patients who normally run on a high blood sugar, a therapeutic trial of glucose is always indicated in diabetics with altered conscious level. Some sulphonylureas (e.g. chlorpropamide) have a long half-life and may cause a late hypoglycaemia even after treatment. Glucagon 0.5–1.0 mg intramuscularly (IM) or slowly IV is an acceptable alternative, although recovery may be slower than with glucose. In resistant cases IV dexamethasone may be used.

Q73
a T b F c F d F e F

Urine testing for ketones is mandatory in all diabetics with hyperglycaemia. Admission in the absence of ketosis or hyperosmolar states is not mandatory and should be reserved for those with difficult control. Hyperkalaemia should not be treated with potassium-lowering agents as the administration of insulin will serve to lower potassium. Supplementation may be needed later. Rapid lowering of blood glucose is not required and may result in rebound hypoglycaemia or cerebral oedema.

Q74
a T b T c T d T e T

The 1993 British Thoracic Society guidelines on the management of asthma include a section on the management of asthma in the A&E department (*Thorax* March 1993 Vol **48** No. 2). They define respiratory failure as a Pao_2 <8 kPa and/or a $Paco_2$ >6 kPa and recommend high flow oxygen for all asthmatics (40–60%). All patients with an initial peak flow less than 50% of that predicted should have arterial blood gases measured. A pulse of ≥110 beats/min and/or a respiratory rate of ≥25 breaths/min indicate severe asthma. IV aminophylline should be considered for those with life threatening features, of which a peak flow <33% predicted is one such feature.

Q75
a F b F c T d T e T

Tension headaches characteristically fail to respond to analgesia and are usually described as tight, constricting, heavy or pressing and experienced on the occiput, vertex or temples. Headache on rising and exacerbated by cough or straining is suggestive of raised intracranial pressure. Scalp tenderness is (rarely) a feature of intracranial neoplasia.

Q76
a T b T c T d F e T

Visual involvement in temporal arteritis is due to an ischaemic optic neuropathy. Ophthalmoplegia can develop due to ischaemic lesions in the third, fourth or sixth cranial nerves. Transient ischaemic attack or stroke may occur if there is involvement of the vertebral or carotid arteries. Pain on eating is a classical sign and is secondary to masseter claudication. A normal ESR does not exclude temporal arteritis and serial ESRs and artery biopsy may be necessary to confirm the diagnosis.

Q77
a F b T c T d F e T

Gout is a disorder of purine metabolism resulting from tissue deposition of crystals of monosodium urate. Acute attacks can occur when the serum urate is normal. The diagnosis may be made using polarized light microscopy of synovial fluid looking for the negatively birefringent crystals of monosodium urate. Treatment in the acute attack consists of rest and use of an NSAID. Colchicine is also effective and characteristically gives dramatic relief from symptoms within a few hours of administration. Its use is now confined to those allergic to NSAIDs because it has a narrow therapeutic index. Allopurinol is used in the prevention of gout but should not be used in the acute phase when it can prolong the attack.

Q78
a F b T c T d T e F

The word migraine means half of the skull. The headache indeed is typically unilateral at onset but may later spread to the whole cranium. Precipitants include physical factors such as bright light or fatigue and dietary agents such as tyramine or monosodium glutamate. Hemiparesis and dysphasia can occasionally accompany the headache and may persist for several days. Ergotamine is effective in 50% of cases but is badly absorbed orally so should be given as a suppository or by inhalation. Migraine is marginally more common in women than men.

Q79
a F **b** F **c** T **d** T **e** T

Hypothermia is defined as a core temperature below 35°C. At this temperature confusion, disorientation and amnesia begin. Semiconsciousness occurs around 33°C and the patient will generally be unconscious with a core temperature of 30°C, when tendon reflexes will be absent. Arrhythmias are common below 33°C but usually spontaneously revert to sinus rhythm on rewarming. Ventricular fibrillation occurs around 28°C and may be precipitated by rough handling. Hypoventilation is a sign of hypothermia and may precede respiratory arrest. The treatment of hypothermia involves careful attention to the airway, breathing and circulation with basic life support continuing until a normal or near normal temperature is achieved.

Q80
a T **b** T **c** F **d** F **e** T

Crescendo angina is differentiated from normal angina by the increased frequency of attacks, failure to respond to normal medication and the presence of reversible ST changes on the ECG. Cardiac enzymes are normal (raised enzymes indicate a myocardial infarction). There is a 15% chance of developing an infarct in the following month; admission is mandatory.

Q81
a F **b** T **c** F **d** T **e** F

ECG signs of right heart strain (SI, QIII and TIII) are uncommon in pulmonary embolus. Linear collapse on chest X-ray is common. Less than 50% of patients with pulmonary embolism have a clinically evident DVT. Pulmonary arteriography is more sensitive – but more invasive – than V/Q scan.

Q82
a T **b** T **c** T **d** F **e** F

Patients who have had a first fit require outpatient follow-up. Admission is not required unless there is a specific reason, for instance, head injury or residual neurological signs.

Q83
a F **b** T **c** F **d** F **e** T

Only 70% of patients who are subsequently proved to have had a myocardial infarction have an abnormal ECG on presentation. Right-sided chest pain may be the presentation of a myocardial infarction due to aberrant myocardial innervation. Linear collapse on a chest X-ray is characteristic of pulmonary embolus, but the chest X-ray is often normal. Urinalysis should always be performed to exclude diabetic ketoacidosis which may present with chest or abdominal pain. Viral costochondritis (usually caused by the coxsackievirus) is a common cause of chest pain and may occur in epidemics.

Q84
a F **b** T **c** T **d** T **e** T

Significant (usually iliofemoral) DVT may be detected by ultrasound but the method is unreliable for below-knee thrombosis, and as clinical diagnosis is unreliable, venography is needed. The treatment of DVT is controversial. All above-knee thromboses require anticoagulation and very large ones may be treated by thrombolysis. The role of anticoagulants in below-knee DVT is not established; all such patients should be referred to the medical admitting team for assessment and follow-up. Where anticoagulation is appropriate, 48 hours of heparin is usually followed by 3 months on warfarin. Homans sign (pain in the calf on dorsiflexing the foot) is positive in DVT but is non-specific and uncomfortable. Its use should be abandoned.

Q85
a F **b** T **c** T **d** F **e** F

Transient ischaemic attacks (TIAs) by definition last less than 24 hours and result from thromboembolism in 90% of cases. Five-year follow-up of TIA patients suggests that 1 in 6 will have a complete stroke and 1 in 4 will have died from stroke or heart disease. Migraine with a focal prodrome or hemiplegic migraine may lead to confusion with TIA, although in the latter a headache is unusual. Carotid TIAs present with aphasia, amaurosis fugax, hemiparesis and hemisensory loss and hemianopic visual disturbance. TIAs of the vertebrobasilar system present with diplopia, vertigo, ataxia, hemisensory loss, hemianopic visual loss, transient global amnesia, and, rarely, loss of consciousness.

Q86
a T **b** T **c** F **d** T **e** T

Subarachnoid haemorrhage results from the rupture of a 'berry' aneurysm in 70% of cases and arteriovenous malformation in 10% of cases. In about 20% of cases no cause is found. Rare associations include bleeding disorders, coarctation of the aorta, Marfan's syndrome and polycystic kidneys. Presentation is usually with sudden headache 'like a blow to the head', with vomiting, although 'warning bleeds' may occur. Initial examination reveals neck stiffness and a positive Kernig's sign and may demonstrate papilloedema, subarachnoid and subretinal haemorrhages. Diagnosis is made by CT scan showing subarachnoid or intraventricular blood. When scanning is not available, lumbar puncture may be performed. There is no evidence to suggest that treatment with dexamethasone is useful, but nimodipine (a calcium channel blocker) has been shown to reduce mortality.

Q87
a F **b** F **c** F **d** F **e** F

Sickle-cell anaemia occurs when the patient is homozygous for the recessive HbS. In the homozygous state more than 80% of the haemoglobin is HbS. Sickle-cell cases arise from either haemolysis or vaso-occlusion (pain crisis). Children may present with the hand-and-foot syndrome with painful swellings of the fingers and toes. Vaso-occlusive disease cases involve bone (the commonest), pleura, brain (hemiparesis or fits), kidney (haematuria), spleen, penis (priapism) and liver. Pain and pyrexia occur, lasting as long as a few days. The Hb level usually remains stable unless aplasia, sequestration of cells in the liver and spleen or haemolysis occurs. The Hb of a sickle-cell-disease patient is usually 6–8 g/dl. Treatment of an acute pain crisis comprises oxygen, IV fluids, analgesia and antibiotics for superadded infection which may precipitate aplasia and haemolysis. Many sickle patients require folate supplements. The commonest precipitant of aplasia is parvovirus infection which may cause simultaneous crisis in more than one affected member of the family.

Multiple choice answers

Resuscitation

Q88
a F b F c F d T e F

The flow through a cannula is proportional to the fourth power of its radius and is inversely proportional to its length. Unless there is no alternative, therefore, central venous cannulae (with low-flow rates) have no role in fluid administration in shock. Their purpose is to measure right heart filling pressure. The internal jugular route is considered safer than the subclavian route which in the emergency situation has a significant iatrogenic pneumothorax rate.

Q89
a T b T c F d F e F

The most direct route for drug administration at a cardiac arrest is via a central line. However, if the personnel present do not have the skill to site a central line rapidly, peripheral cannulation should take place. The intraosseous route is useful in children and the endotracheal route can be used if all else fails. Opioid analgesics have no place in the early management of the arrested patient but may be needed later if the resuscitation is successful. Defibrillation should only be used in those patients with ventricular fibrillation and those in whom the diagnosis of ventricular fibrillation cannot be excluded. Adrenaline and atropine both affect pupillary size so the pupils should not be used as an indicator of when to stop resuscitation.

Q90
a F b F c T d T e T

Atropine 3 mg is given only in the management of asystole. Calcium chloride is only indicated if EMD is thought to be due to calcium channel blocker overdose. High-dose adrenaline should be considered if the arrest is prolonged. Successful treatment of EMD depends on the recognition of its cause. In children this is most commonly hypovolaemia and a bolus of 20 ml/kg of fluid intravenously or intraosseously is therefore included in the paediatric algorithm. If cardiac tamponade is suspected, a pericardiocentesis should be performed. Other causes of EMD include tension pneumothorax, pulmonary embolism, drugs, hypothermia and electrolyte imbalance.

Q91
a T b F c T d F e F

In this situation a precordial thump should be tried. If this fails, electrical cardioversion should begin, starting at 200 J. Synchronized shock should not be used as the defibrillator will not be able to find an 'R' wave. After two further shocks (200 then 360 J), basic life support (if not previously instituted) should commence. 10 ml of adrenaline 1:10 000 is then given intravenously. Atropine is not used in a cardiac arrest secondary to ventricular fibrillation. The prognosis of cardiac arrest with ventricular fibrillation is much better than if the rhythm is asystole.

Q92
a F b T c T d T e T

Asystolic arrest occurs when there is no ventricular activity. 'P' waves may be present. Adrenaline 1 mg should be given and repeated every 2–3 minutes. Atropine may be used once only in a dose of 3 mg. If there are any signs of electrical activity, pacing should be considered. Asystole is the commonest arrest rhythm in children, as a progression of the bradycardia that occurs with severe hypoxia.

Q93
a T b T c T d F e F

The causes of electromechanical dissociation include hypovolaemia, hypothermia, pulmonary embolus, cardiac tamponade, tension pneumothorax and electrolyte imbalance. Drugs which are negatively inotropic such as the β-blockers, calcium antagonists and lignocaine can also be responsible. Ketamine will increase the blood pressure and is the anaesthetic agent of choice in the shocked patient.

Q94
a F **b** T **c** F **d** T **e** T

Lignocaine decreases ventricular automaticity through its class 1B antiarrhythmic effect and suppresses ectopics through its local anaesthetic effect. The threshold for ventricular fibrillation is increased, but so is the energy required for successful defibrillation. Torsade de pointes should be treated by correcting the underlying cause (e.g. electrolyte disorders) rather than by the use of antiarrhythmics (lignocaine is contraindicated). Bretylium is an adrenergic neuron-blocking agent and takes about 20 minutes to become effective.

Q95
a F **b** F **c** F **d** F **e** T

Adrenaline is one of the most useful drugs available to the emergency physician. It is a directly acting sympathomimetic amine with both α- and β-adrenergic activity. It should be given intravenously at cardiac arrest in a dose of 1 mg every 2–3 minutes. The endotracheal route can be used if cannulation is not possible. The dosage should then be doubled. Adrenaline can also be given intramuscularly. This is the route that patients with atopic anaphylaxis use for self-injection. Adrenaline should not be mixed with lignocaine for digital blocks as it may cause vasoconstriction in an end artery and subsequent digital ischaemia.

Q96
a T **b** T **c** T **d** T **e** F

The use of sodium bicarbonate in cardiac arrest in adults has gone out of favour. If given, it produces hyperosmolality, hypernatraemia and generates large amounts of carbon dioxide. This diffuses into cells, exacerbating the intracellular acidosis. It may sometimes be indicated in patients with a pre-existing metabolic acidosis. In these cases it should be given in a dose of 1 mmol/kg. 1 ml of 8.4% solution contains 1 mmol. Care should be taken when it is infused, as extravasation may result in severe tissue ulceration.

Q97
a F b F c T d F e T

Laryngeal masks do not provide adequate protection against aspiration. They have the advantage of being simple to insert but their use in resuscitation has not yet been fully evaluated. A guide can be passed down the tube of the mask into the trachea, and an endotracheal tube can then be railroaded over the guide following removal of the mask.

Q98
a T b T c F d T e T

The formula for endotracheal tube diameter is

$$\frac{age\ (in\ years)}{4} + 4$$

or approximately the diameter of the patient's little finger or width of the nostril.

Q99
a T b T c T d F e F

Open cardiac massage may allow control of haemorrhage and is therefore indicated in cardiac arrest due to hypovolaemia secondary to penetrating cardiac trauma. It produces a significantly higher cardiac output than closed massage (up to 2.5 times greater in animal studies). In the emergency situation it is carried out through a left lower thoracotomy. Extensive laboratory and limited clinical studies suggest higher survival rates for open compression. Other suggested indications include patients with a recent sternotomy and patients in whom closed compressions are likely to be unsuccessful for physical reasons such as emphysema. (Compression techniques and bloodflow during cardiopulmonary resuscitation. *Resuscitation* **24** (1992): 123–132).

Q100
a T b T c F d F e T

Lignocaine (Vaughan Williams classification Ib), which reduces the entry of sodium into cells and therefore stabilizes the cell membrane, is ineffective at low temperatures and when given by the endotracheal route. Lignocaine 100 mg IV is appropriate for the treatment of ventricular tachycardia where cardiac output is present.

Q101
a T **b** F **c** T **d** T **e** T

Atrioventricular dissociation, fusion beats, capture beats, QRS duration > 0.14 seconds, a deep S wave in V6 and concordant QRS direction in all chest leads are all suggestive of VT. Availability of a previous ECG may reveal a long-standing left bundle branch block, suggesting the possibility of SVT with aberrant conduction as a cause of a broad complex tachycardia.

Q102
a T **b** T **c** F **d** T **e** F

Supraventricular tachycardias are associated with caffeine intake, Wolff–Parkinson–White syndrome and other accessory pathways. If resolution does not follow a vagotonic manoeuvre such as carotid sinus massage, adenosine should be given. Over 90% of supraventricular tachycardias will respond. Verapamil is also very effective but, as it is negatively inotropic, it should be avoided if the blood pressure is low. Adrenaline will worsen the arrhythmia and should not be used.

Q103
a T **b** F **c** F **d** F **e** F

Type I second-degree heart block (Wenckebach) is characterized by an increasing PR interval, followed by a dropped beat and recovery of the PR interval and a repeat of the cycle. This is a transient arrhythmia and is considered to be benign. In type II second-degree heart block there is intermittent non-conduction of some P waves, but the PR interval is constant. This arrhythmia may progress to ventricular dysrhythmias or asystole. In third-degree heart block the RR interval is constant if there is a single ventricular pacemaker.

Q104
a F b T c T d T e T

Complete heart block leads to total dissociation between the atria and ventricles; the PR interval is therefore variable. The rate depends on the site of the ventricular pacemaker: rates of 50 result from pacemakers near the atrioventricular node, rates of 40 result from more distal pacemakers. Hypotension may occur and may be the cause of the patient's presentation. Atropine may improve the rate in the short term, but pacing is usually required.

Overdose and substance abuse

Q105
a T b T c T d F e T

The most important side-effects of tricyclic antidepressants are arrhythmias and convulsions. Drowsiness, coma, hypotension, hypertension, hyperthermia, hyperreflexia, dilated pupils and urinary retention also occur. Treatment is supportive with intravenous diazepam for convulsions.

Q106
a T b T c T d F e T

Mefenamic acid (Ponstan) is a non-steroidal anti-inflammatory analgesic which inhibits prostaglandin activity. Complications of overdosage include: diarrhoea, rashes, drowsiness, dizziness and acute renal failure. Treatment is supportive with administration of activated charcoal and monitoring of renal function.

Q107
a F b T c T d F e F

Gastric lavage is of no value in the treatment of benzodiazepine overdose, for which the specific antidote is flumazenil (Anexate). Hostile behaviour and confusion occur in a proportion of patients taking benzodiazepines. Because of problems with addiction, benzodiazepines can now only be recommended for occasional use in acute anxiety states. Insomnia, anxiety, loss of appetite, tremor, perspiration and tinnitus occur on withdrawal.

Multiple choice answers

Q108
a T b T c T d F e T

Aspirin overdose commonly causes tinnitus, deafness, nausea and vomiting. Central nervous system features such as coma and convulsions are a feature of more severe poisoning. Acid–base balance is influenced by two confounding effects. Direct stimulation of the respiratory centre causes a respiratory alkalosis whilst uncoupling of oxidative phosphorylation results in metabolic acidosis. In young children the metabolic component usually dominates. Mild cases may be treated by increasing the oral fluid intake. In more severe cases activated charcoal should be used. It significantly shortens the plasma half-life of salicylates. Urine alkalinization using intravenous sodium bicarbonate hastens the excretion of the weakly acidic salicylates and may also be considered.

Q109
a T b T c T d T e T

Co-proxamol is a combination analgesic containing paracetamol and dextropropoxyphene. If taken in overdose the opiate will cause respiratory depression and paracetamol will cause liver failure. The respiratory depression can be reversed with naloxone. If the paracetamol level is below the treatment threshold, opiate levels will also be low and the overdose will not require any clinical intervention.

Q110
a T b T c T d T e T

Solvent abuse (e.g. petroleum-based solvents, halogenated hydrocarbons and butane) causes confusion, convulsions, euphoria, hallucinations, headache, psychosis, arrhythmias, ataxia, drooling, hypotension, peripheral neuropathy, renal failure, cardiac arrest, DIC, hypokalaemia and methaemoglobinaemia.

Q111
a F **b** T **c** T **d** T **e** T

Cannabis, the Indian hemp plant, is usually smoked or ingested. If smoked the effects start within 10–20 minutes and last up to 3 hours. Symptoms are very variable but include mild anxiety followed by a period of calm. An irritating cough may occur and perception of colour and sound is often enhanced. Injection of the drug can lead to coma and precipitate myocardial ischaemia.

Q112
a F **b** T **c** T **d** T **e** T

Fifty per cent of alcoholics have a normal liver. Although there are many behavioural and psychiatric manifestations of alcohol abuse, true Wernicke's encephalopathy is rare. Disulfiram is Antabuse.

Q113
a T **b** T **c** F **d** T **e** T

Stimulant abuse (e.g. amphetamine, amphetamine-like antiobesity drugs, Ecstasy and caffeine) causes agitation, anxiety, hallucinations, hyperactivity, paranoia, arrhythmias, coma, convulsion, dilated pupils, hypertension, hyperpyrexia, hyperventilation, stroke and myocardial infarction.

Q114
a F **b** F **c** F **d** T **e** F

Carboxyhaemoglobin levels correlate poorly with severity of poisoning. It is the plasma carbon monoxide (CO) level and the mitochondrial enzyme levels which reflect the severity. Patients show benefit from hyperbaric oxygen therapy even several days after exposure. This is because of the long half-life of CO–respiratory enzyme complexes. Any patient with symptoms of CO poisoning, no matter how long after exposure, should be discussed with the nearest hyperbaric unit. Cardiac failure is a positive indication for hyperbaric therapy. Metabolic acidosis is a feature of CO poisoning. 'Cherry-red' lips are an uncommon finding.

Multiple choice answers

Q115
a T b T c T d F e F

Amyl nitrite induces the production of methaemoglobin.
Cobalt-EDTA is a specific antidote for cyanide and acts by direct
chelation. It is, however, very toxic and may cause anaphylaxis. For
this reason it should only be used when poisoning is certain. Cyanide
assays are not generally available outside specialist centres.

Q116
a F b T c F d F e T

Only one death from laburnum poisoning has been reported in the
UK in the last 50 years. Symptomatic poisonings are rare, but
symptoms include drowsiness, twitching, convulsions, nausea and
vomiting. The value of gastric lavage is doubtful, although it may be
indicated in severe poisoning. Routine admission is not required.

Q117
a F b T c F d F e T

Paraquat is a 'total' weedkiller which is fatal on ingestion (with
doses of 10 ml of a 20% solution or more). Multiple organ failure
following overdose usually occurs within 6–48 hours of exposure.
Gastric lavage followed by Fuller's earth, bentonite or activated
charcoal instillation repeated 4-hourly is effective in reducing
absorption. Prognosis can be predicted from serum levels by
comparison with an appropriate nomogram. Skin contamination
usually results in blistering, ulceration and irritation only.

Q118
a T b T c T d T e T

Naloxone is a specific opioid antagonist. It is usually given by
intravenous administration. If venous access is not possible the
intramuscular route may be used. It is effective within 2 minutes of
administration but has a short half-life. An intravenous infusion is
therefore an effective way of administering the drug. It has a wide
therapeutic index and low incidence of adverse effects. High doses
may be needed to reverse serious opiate overdosage.

Q119
a T **b** F **c** F **d** F **e** T

Flumazenil is a benzodiazepine antagonist and will reverse the toxic
effects of these drugs within a minute. It has a half-life of an hour so
infusions may be necessary. Doses of more than 1 mg can be given
but failure to respond after 5 mg virtually excludes benzodiazepines
as a cause of coma. Side-effects include severe hypotension,
dysrhythmias and convulsions which may be difficult to control. For
these reasons it is not yet recommended for routine use as a
diagnostic test in unconscious patients.

Q120
a T **b** F **c** T **d** T **e** F

The phenothiazines and butyrophenones are both causes of dystonic
reactions. Procyclidine is used for treatment of these conditions.
Cimetidine can cause confusion but is not associated with oculogyric
crisis.

Infectious diseases

Q121
a F **b** F **c** F **d** T **e** F

The herald patch of pityriasis rosea usually occurs a few days before
the appearance of the characteristic widespread itchy rash which lasts
a further 4–6 weeks. Erysipelas is a skin infection caused by
Streptococcus pyogenes. The description in (c) is that of psoriasis.
After an incubation period of 10 days, measles begins with fever,
coryza and small white Koplik's spots on the buccal mucosa. The
characteristic maculopapular rash begins on the neck spreading to the
face, trunks and limbs.

The pink macular rash of rubella normally lasts 2–3 days, often
becoming confluent on the trunk. The incubation period is about 18
days.

Q122
a T b F c T d F e T

Erysipelas is an erythematous rash which characteristically has a sharply demarcated and palpable edge. It is commonest at the extremes of age and usually affects the face or legs. The rash of varicella is first maculopapular then vesicular before it begins to crust. The rash of rubella consists of discrete pink macules. These appear first on the face and then spread downwards. Erythema marginatum is associated with acute rheumatic fever or drug reactions and not with any infective agents.

Q123
a F b F c F d F e F

Malaria may present at any time up to several years after initial exposure. Diagnosis is by thick and thin blood films, which may have to be repeated on several occasions to observe parasites. Prophylaxis reduces the probability that a person will contract malaria, but does not exclude the diagnosis. Cases of malaria arising in people who have not travelled abroad but who live near to airports have been reported. Cerebral malaria is a medical emergency and should be treated prior to transfer.

Q124
a F b T c F d T e T

Fatal chickenpox pneumonitis has been reported in pregnant women and those on steroids. Suspected cases should be admitted to hospital. Acyclovir is effective if used early and reduces the duration and severity of the attack as well as the severity of postherpetic neuralgia. Shingles cannot be caught from a patient with shingles but chickenpox can!

Q125
a F b T c T d F e T

The mite causing scabies is an arachnid, *Sarcoptes scabiei*. The young are more prone to infestation than the old. Itching may increase in severity for up to 2 weeks following treatment.

Q126
a T b T c T d T e T

PUO is defined as a fever lasting for more than 14 days without a cause being found.

Q127
a F b T c T d T e F

HIV-positive patients may remain symptom-free for 10 or more years after diagnosis. The diagnosis of AIDS relies upon identifying positive characteristic clinical manifestations of the disease in patients with certain defined infections. The finding of a CD4 count of less than 200×10^6 in the presence of HIV-positive status is however diagnostic, even in the absence of clinical signs of AIDS. AIDs or HIV-positive patients should generally be nursed in open wards. Tetanus toxoid is not contraindicated.

Q128
a T b T c F d F e T

Hepatitis A can now be prevented by active immunization with a vaccine but normal immunoglobulin should be added for postexposure prophylaxis. There have not been any reported cases of hepatitis B following mouth-to-mouth ventilation. Use of a handkerchief as a barrier is not considered effective and may actually increase the risk of virus transmission. A positive e antigen indicates a high risk of infectivity. Hepatitis C is usually transmitted by the blood-borne route. All blood donations in the UK are now screened for this virus.

Q129
a T b T c T d T e T

All patients with suspected meningococcal septicaemia/meningitis should have benzylpenicillin administered parenterally by the first attending physician.

Psychiatry

Q130
a T b T c T d T e T

Those likely to succeed in a suicide attempt include the elderly, particularly males, the single, unemployed, those with mental illness or severe physical illness and those who abuse drugs or alcohol. The suicide rate for doctors is approximately three times that for the general population, partially related to the higher level of alcohol abuse.

Q131
a F b T c F d F e T

Section 2 of the Mental Health Act 1983 allows admission for up to 28 days for assessment following application by an approved social worker or nearest relative and recommendation by two doctors, one of whom must be approved under the act. Section 3 allows admission for treatment for up to 6 months. Section 4 allows admission for up to 72 hours in an emergency after assessment by a social worker and a doctor not approved under the act and should be converted to a section 2 as soon as possible. Under section 136 police officers have the power to remove from a public place to a place of safety persons who appear to be suffering from a mental disorder either in that patient's own interests or for the protection of others. A police station or a hospital casualty department is a place of safety under the act. The Mental Health Act does not apply to persons who are intoxicated by alcohol or drugs. The patient threatening suicide may be admitted under the Mental Health Act only if suffering from a recognized psychiatric disorder. Restraint under common law may also be considered.

Q132
a T b T c T d T e T

The list should also include tricyclic antidepressants, anticonvulsants, antiarrhythmics and digoxin. A detailed drug history may be very relevant in these patients.

Q133
a T b T c F d T e T

Parasuicide is more common in women, whilst completed suicide is more common in men. All patients who present to the A&E department with attempted suicide should have a mental state examination performed. In 1984 the Department of Health decided that some screening of admission should take place so not all patients need to be admitted. The SAD PERSONS scale is a scoring system that can be used to assess the need for hospitalization of this group.

Q134
a F b T c T d F e F

A potentially violent patient should be assessed in a room where there is no loose furniture. You must make sure that you have a clear avenue of exit and that help is available right outside the room. Crockery can be used as a weapon so should not be offered. Avoid looking the patient in the eye as this is seen as a sign of challenge. If you need to restrain a patient, six or more people will be needed (one for each arm and two for each leg).

Q135
a T b F c T d T e F

Visual hallucinations tend to point to an organic pathology, whilst auditory hallucinations are usually due to a functional cause. Other indicators of an organic cause are sudden-onset impairment of recent memory, emotional lability, hyper- or hypoactivity and ataxia.

Multiple choice answers

Surgery

Q136
a T b T c T d T e T

Ten per cent of gallstones are visible on plain abdominal X-ray, by virtue of calcification within the stone. One or both psoas shadows may be obliterated by the presence of free fluid in the abdomen or retroperitoneal space. Dilated loops of bowel are a feature of obstruction on the supine film. On the erect film obstruction is characterized by fluid levels. Subdiaphragmatic gas develops with a perforated viscus, but can also be seen after insufflation of carbon dioxide for laparoscopy. The outline of an enlarged spleen may sometimes be visible extending from the left upper quadrant towards the right lower quadrant.

Q137
a T b T c T d T e F

The commonest cause of pancreatitis in the UK is biliary tract disease. Mild jaundice, probably obstructive in origin, may be an early feature. Low serum calcium is a poor prognostic feature. Both serum and urine will show elevated amylase. Pethidine is the analgesic of choice.

Q138
a T b T c T d T e T

The commonest presentation of testicular torsion is sudden onset of groin and lower abdominal pain and vomiting, although vomiting alone may occur. Inflammation of the scrotum follows and may mimic epididymo-orchitis. A mild pyrexia is usual.

Q139
a T b F c F d T e F

NSAIDs are the analgesic of choice for the treatment of pain of renal colic. Pethidine is indicated if NSAIDs are contraindicated. Haematuria is present in about 90% of cases of renal colic and 90% of stones are visible on the plain abdominal film. Vomiting is a feature of renal colic. IV antibiotics are not generally required unless there is evidence of infection. If there is evidence of sepsis in the presence of an obstructed kidney, urgent urological intervention is required to relieve the obstruction.

90

Q140
a T b F c T d T e T

Small-bowel obstruction most commonly occurs from adhesions, long after the original surgery. An obturator hernia should be suspected in the elderly female presenting with bowel obstruction and a painful thigh. Femoral hernias have a tight neck and frequently obstruct. All patients with intestinal obstruction should be treated with intravenous fluids and a nasogastric tube to aspirate stomach contents.

Q141
a F b F c F d T e F

Pyloric stenosis is about four times more common in boys than girls. It presents in the first month of life with projectile, non-bile-stained vomitus. Diagnosis is clinical and is confirmed by ultrasound. Emergency surgery is not indicated; the emphasis is upon adequate resuscitation followed by urgent surgery.

Q142
a T b T c T d T e T

Intussusception is most common in children under the age of 2 years. The incidence is higher in Negroes and those from the Far East rather than in Caucasians. The presence of a sausage-shaped abdominal mass, redcurrant jelly stool or a characteristic shadow on the plain abdominal X-ray all suggest the diagnosis. In early intussusception (<24 hours), reduction by barium enema may be achieved.

Paediatrics

Q143
a F b F c T d F e T

The anterior fontanelle usually closes in the middle of the second year. Although a sunken fontanelle indicates marked dehydration, the fontanelle is not a sensitive indicator of fluid status. The commonest cause of a bulging fontanelle is a crying infant.

Q144
a F b T c F d T e F

The diagnosis of acute epiglottitis is made from the history and clinical appearance. Once made, the child should be admitted immediately without further investigation. Careful induction of anaesthetic and intubation by a senior anaesthetist will be required. Any attempt at intubation, laryngoscopy, IV access and even application of an oxygen mask may precipitate complete airway obstruction. The onset of epiglottitis is rapid with no preceding coryza and only slight cough. The child is characteristically toxic, with a temperature greater than 38.5°C and drools saliva. Croup, in comparison, presents with a longer history, a severe cough and moderate pyrexia. Stridor is harsh and there is no drooling.

Q145
a F b T c T d F e F

Gastroenteritis produced by organisms that invade the mucosa such as *Salmonella* and *Shigella* tends to cause bloody mucoid stools. If produced by enterotoxin forming organisms such as *Staphylococcus aureus* the diarrhoea tends to be watery. Egg products and poultry are the common sources of *Salmonella* poisoning. Antibiotics should not be given as they can prolong the shedding of the organism. Treatment of the condition centres around rehydration. Babies should only be discharged if adequately hydrated and when proper follow-up is in place. Diphenoxylate can precipitate toxic megacolon if given to patients with invasive diarrhoea and so should be avoided.

Q146
a T b F c T d T e F

Non-accidental injury is most common in those under the age of 1 but can occur at any age. Subdural haematomas and retinal haemorrhages are secondary to shaking. Epiphyseal separation is caused by swinging the child. Pretibial bruising and fractured clavicle are common injuries and are not usually associated with child abuse. The paediatric team should be called whenever the diagnosis is suspected.

Q147
a F b T c F d F e F

Meningitis in children may not present in the classically described manner, particularly in children under the age of 18 months. A bulging fontanelle, failure to feed, irritability and drowsiness may be the only signs. Papilloedema is a late sign of raised intracranial pressure and cannot reliably be used to exclude the diagnosis. In all cases of suspected meningitis, IV benzylpenicillin should be given by the first doctor to see the child. Delay to establish the diagnosis by lumbar puncture may prove fatal. Meningococcal meningitis has a rapid onset and may progress to death within 12–24 hours, *Haemophilus* meningitis has a more insidious onset and the diagnosis is frequently delayed.

Q148
a F b T c T d F e F

Febrile fits are defined as a symmetrical tonic/clonic seizure in a child between the age of 3 months and 5 years occurring in the presence of a temperature. The temperature may be normal on presentation to hospital, although there is usually a history of a viral illness. Focal fits and fits in children under 3 months or over 5 years should lead to the search for other pathology.

Q149
a T b T c T d T e T

All of the mentioned features suggest the possibility of non-accidental injury. The actual diagnosis must be made by a senior paediatrician in conjunction with social services and possibly the police. All suspected cases must therefore be referred for an expert opinion.

Q150
a T b T c T d F e T

Dysuria in children is often associated with sterile urine. Children with urinary tract infections present in non-specific way, e.g. gastroenteritis, failure to thrive or septicaemia.

Multiple choice answers

Q151
a T b F c F d T e T

Q152
a F b T c T d F e F

Croup is characterized by a slow onset over several days, often preceded by a coryzal illness. An intermittent harsh stridor, hoarse voice and barking cough are common. The child may be apyrexial or have a low fever.

Q153
a F b T c F d T e F

Child sexual abuse is becoming increasingly recognized but remains a very complex clinical problem. If the diagnosis is suspected the child should be immediately referred to the paediatric unit. Confirmation may need extensive investigation and careful examination by a multidisciplinary team. It is more common in girls than boys and the offenders are the parents or guardian in around 50% of the cases. Reflex anal dilatation in children is abnormal and suspicious and requires further investigation but is not pathognomomonic of anal abuse (Cleveland inquiry, 1988). Other signs of sexual abuse include palatal petechiae, scarring of the hymen and venereal disease.

Q154
a T b T c F d F e T

Acute asthma is the commonest reason for hospital admission of a child in the UK. The incidence of asthma continues to rise in the community. Peak flow is a reliable measurement of severity but is difficult to measure accurately in young children. Chest X-ray is only indicated if there are signs of severe infection, pneumothorax or if the diagnosis is in doubt. Steroids should be given orally unless the child is vomiting. Increased secretion of antidiuretic hormone in severe asthma can result in fluid retention, so fluid intake should be restricted to two-thirds of normal.

Q155
a F b T c F d F e T

The basic fluid requirements of a child can be worked out as follows: for the first 10 kg of weight the child needs 100 ml/kg, for the second 10 kg 50 ml and for each subsequent kilogram, 20 ml. The requirement of this child is therefore 1540 ml. A decreased urine output is an early sign of dehydration but drowsiness will only occur with moderate to severe fluid deficit. Fluid replacement in the dehydrated child should commence with 0.45% saline and dextrose. Further therapy then depends on the serum sodium. The shocked child can receive 20 ml/kg of crystalloid or colloid before reassessment. If there is no change a second bolus should be given. If there is still no response an urgent surgical opinion should be sought.

Q156
a T b F c F d T e F

Respiratory syncyitial virus is the cause of 75% of the cases of bronchiolitis. Epidemics occur in the winter and affect children in their first year. Treatment is non-specific with humidified oxygen. Antibiotics, steroids and bronchodilators are of no proved value. The antiviral agent ribavirin is used in more severe cases.

Gynaecology

Q157
a F b F c F d T e T

One in 500 pregnancies in the UK develop in a site other than the uterus. There is an increased risk of ectopic pregnancy following pelvic inflammatory disease and tubal surgery, in those who use an intrauterine contraceptive device and in those taking the progesterone-only pill. Ruptured ectopic pregnancy characteristically presents around the time of the first missed period with pelvic and lower abdominal pain. There may be a slight dark red vaginal loss. Haemodynamic collapse can ensue rapidly. The diagnosis should be clinical and urgent laparotomy is required. Delay must not be allowed to occur whilst biochemical or ultrasound confirmation is obtained. If the diagnosis of ruptured ectopic pregnancy is in doubt and the patient is haemodynamically stable then ultrasound examination may be appropriate. Following surgery for ectopic pregnancy, there is a 10% chance of further ectopic pregnancy in the other fallopian tube, with each subsequent conception.

Q158
a T **b** F **c** T **d** T **e** T

The morning-after pill frequently causes vomiting. If this occurs within 2 hours of ingestion, consideration should be given to the taking of another pill. It is effective if taken within 72 hours of unprotected intercourse. The efficacy may however be reduced by concomitant administration of antibiotics such as ampicillin and griseofulvin, barbiturates and phenytoin. It is contraindicated in patients with a clotting disorder and should not be used if the patient has a confirmed pregnancy.

Q159
a T **b** T **c** F **d** T **e** T

Placental abruption is characterized by abdominal pain and tenderness localized to the uterus. Placenta praevia does not usually cause pain. Both acute appendicitis in pregnancy and pre-eclampsia can cause right upper quadrant pain. With appendicitis this is due to the higher position of the inflamed appendix, whereas with pre-eclampsia it is secondary to the stretched capsule of the engorged liver.

Q160
a F **b** T **c** T **d** T **e** F

Associations with ectopic pregnancy include pelvic inflammatory disease, tubal surgery, the intrauterine contraceptive device and the progesterone-only pill. The home pregnancy test may be negative in cases of ectopic pregnancy. A blood test or sensitive urine analysis is necessary to exclude the diagnosis. Ectopic pregnancy cannot be felt bimanually.

Q161
a T b F c T d F e F

Pre-eclampsia is characterized by a blood pressure elevation of more than 30 mmHg over booking blood pressure. Oedema may or may not occur. Proteinuria is a late sign and indicates renal involvement. Liver involvement leads to DIC. Untreated, it may progress to fits (eclampsia) and lead to maternal death from stroke, renal, liver or cardiac failure. Pre-eclampsia may resemble a viral illness, with fever, headache, tachycardia. Other symptoms include chest or epigastric pain, vomiting, visual disturbances, irritability, and later papilloedema. All pregnant women should have their blood pressure measured, urinalysis performed and be examined for oedema; any signs of pre-eclampsia warrant urgent obstetric referral.

Q162
a T b T c T d T e F

Cord prolapse is an obstetric emergency; early prompt treatment to prevent fetal asphyxia followed by caesarean section may be life saving. Cord compression leads to fetal asphyxia. The 'first aid' treatment is therefore to prevent the presenting part occluding the cord. It should be displaced upwards towards the mother's head using a hand in the vagina. The mother may be placed in the knee–elbow position (kneeling so the rump is higher than the head), using gravity to displace the presenting part. The cord should not be handled, as spasm may occur. The definitive treatment is a caesarean section or forceps delivery if the cervix is fully dilated.

Q163
a T b F c T d T e T

APH is defined as vaginal bleeding occurring after 28 weeks' gestation. The causes include placental abruption, placenta praevia (hence vaginal examination should not be performed), cervical polyps and cervicitis. Severe bleeding may be complicated by DIC due to thromboplastin release. Anti-D immunoglobulin should be given as soon as possible to susceptible women (250 IU <20 weeks' gestation, 500 IU >20 weeks' gestation).

Q164
a T **b** F **c** F **d** T **e** T

PPH may be primary or secondary. Primary PPH occurs in the first 24 hours after delivery and is caused by uterine atony (90%), genital tract trauma and clotting disorders. Initial management includes basic resuscitation and administration of ergotamine 0.5 mg IV. If bleeding continues, oxytocin 10 units in 500 ml dextrose at a rate of 15 drops/minute should be given. Expert obstetric help should be sought early. Secondary PPH is bleeding from the genital tract more than 24 hours after delivery (usually 5–12 days). It is caused by retained products of conception, clot or secondary infection. Antibiotics should be given if there is evidence of infection. Retained products or clot should be removed by dilatation and curettage.

Q165
a T **b** F **c** T **d** F **e** T

Pelvic inflammatory disease is usually acquired through sexual contact (90%). The diagnosis is often made on laparoscopy; clinical diagnosis may detect only 30% of cases. Because of the need to culture for sexually transmitted organisms, the treatment is best carried out by those experienced in this field – either genitourinary physicians or gynaecologists. Treatment in the A&E department is not warranted as a positive diagnosis of the causative organism may not be made and contact tracing is often not initiated. In severe cases admission may be required for IV antibiotics. Failure to treat this condition adequately can lead to infertility or ectopic pregnancy.

Ear, nose and throat

Q166
a F **b** T **c** F **d** F **e** T

Control of epistaxis is achieved by compression of the soft part of the nose. If a nasal pack is inserted it should be removed after 24 hours. There is no need to check a full blood count routinely after a nose bleed. Patients who have suffered blunt nasal trauma should be warned that they should expect slight epistaxis following the injury which is of no significance.

Q167
a T b T c T d F e F

Quinsy (peritonsillar abscess) is usually unilateral, although contralateral involvement may develop a few days after the original presentation. Dysphagia is characteristic, often leading to dribbling of saliva. It is more common in adult males and is treated by incision and drainage under local anaesthetic.

Q168
a T b T c F d F e F

A subperichondrial haematoma is caused by shearing blows to the ear. The perichondrium is stripped from the cartilage by the haematoma. If the patient is seen acutely the blood should be aspirated and a pressure dressing applied. Surgical drainage is necessary if the haematoma is more chronic. A cauliflower ear occurs when the cartilage collapses. This can be precipitated by a subperichondrial haematoma or by infection.

Q169
a T b T c F d T e F

Mercury batteries that lodge in the oesophagus or fail to leave the stomach must be removed as a matter of urgency. X-ray examination may fail to show radiolucent foreign bodies or fish bones. Patients with suspected bones in their throat must undergo indirect laryngoscopy.

Q170
a T b F c T d T e T

There is no evidence that steroids alter the duration or outcome of Bell's palsy, although some centres advocate their use.

Ophthalmology

Q171
a T b T c F d F e T

The pupil in Holmes–Adie syndrome is dilated and fails to react to light or reacts very slowly. During accommodation it constricts very slowly. A complete third-nerve palsy causes ptosis and a fixed down and out position of the eye as well as pupillary dilatation. Myasthenia gravis causes ptosis but not pupillary changes. The ipsilateral pupil in a Horner's syndrome is constricted so the contralateral pupil will appear dilated.

Q172
a F b T c T d T e T

Pupillary constriction is an early sign of organophosphate poisoning (remember that the initial treatment is with high-dose atropine). A unilateral dilated pupil may be found after an epileptic fit but the possibility of a fit secondary to a serious head injury should not be ignored. Small pupils (senile miosis) are a common feature in old age. Both atropine and adrenaline cause pupillary dilatation, hence fixed dilated pupils are an invalid sign following treated cardiac arrest.

Q173
a F b F c T d F e T

Treatment of metallic corneal foreign bodies includes a careful history to determine whether a high- or low-velocity foreign body is involved, inspection of the cornea, conjunctiva and under both lids using a local anaesthetic such as amethocaine. Patching is not usually necessary following the use of such short acting agents. Fluorescein should be used routinely to demonstrate corneal abrasions and patients with corneal rust staining should be referred for an ophthalmological opinion. Orbital X-rays are required if there is any possibility of penetrating foreign body.

Q174
a T b F c T d F e T

The patient should be nursed on his or her back to avoid adhesion of
the iris to the cornea and production of anterior synechiae. Similarly,
anything causing raised intraocular pressure (coughing, straining and
pressure measurement) should be avoided to prevent extrusion of
ocular contents. Penetrating injuries may produce either an irregular
pupil or a fixed dilated pupil.

Q175
a T b T c F d T e F

Formal assessment of visual acuity with a Snellen chart is an
essential component of the examination of every patient who presents
to the A&E department with an eye problem. Fluorescein should be
used to demonstrate corneal abrasions but topical anaesthetics impair
corneal healing and a single application only is indicated. Alkali
continues to damage the eye after the initial contamination and urgent
referral is appropriate after copious lavage. Neither acid nor alkali
should be neutralized, as this produces heat and provides further
damage, but rather lavaged with copious amounts of normal saline
(500–1000 ml per eye).

Q176
a F b T c F d T e F

Atropine, when instilled in the eye, causes very long acting (up to 2
weeks) pupillary dilatation which is difficult to reverse. Other, more
short-acting agents such as tropicamide or homatropine should be
used in the A&E department. Phenylephrine is a sympathomimetic
agent which causes pupillary dilatation. It should be avoided in
patients with cardiac disease. Fluorescein is a corneal stain, whilst
Rose Bengal stains damaged conjunctival or corneal epithelium.
Topical acyclovir ointment 3% five times a day is the treatment of
choice for a dendritic ulcer. The use of steroid eye drops should be
avoided in the A&E department as they may provoke worsening of
infective eye conditions, particularly an unexpected herpetic dendritic
ulcer.

Q177
a T b F c F d F e F

Visual disturbance is one of the cardinal symptoms of pathology in the eye. Visual acuity should be checked in all patients who attend the A&E department with symptoms related to the eye. Acute closed-angle glaucoma occurs in patients with a shallow anterior chamber. Poor drainage causes rising intraocular pressure and an oedematous cornea. This results in clouding of vision. A damaged lens becomes opaque resulting in a cataract, but onset is not usually sudden. The only symptom may be visual disturbance. The absence of visual symptoms is usually good confirmatory evidence of a diagnosis of conjunctivitis in a patient with a red eye. Episcleritis is a painful inflammatory nodule often associated with rheumatic disorders.

Q178
a F b F c T d T e T

Snow blindness and arc eye both result from ultraviolet exposure and are usually bilateral. They may cause short-term visual impairment. They characteristically produce a 'starry night' appearance on corneal staining due to multiple small erosions. First-aid treatment should include oral analgesics and taping of the eye closed. Regular topical anaesthetics can hinder the regeneration of the conjunctival epithelium.

Q179
a T b T c F d T e T

Orbital cellulitis can follow trauma or spread of infection from blood, the sinuses or the skin. The most common causative organism is *Staphylococcus aureus*, followed by *Haemophilus influenzae*, *Streptococcus pneumoniae* and the anaerobes. Decreased ocular motility and tenderness upon eye movement are characteristic. There may be decreased sensation in the area of the ophthalmic and maxillary branches of the trigeminal nerve. Spread of infection to the facial venous system and subsequent cavernous sinus thrombosis must be prevented. Intravenous antibiotics, usually an antistaphylococcal agent and a cephalosporin should be used.

Q180
a T b T c F d T e T

Retinal detachment is more common in the myopic eye. It may be primary idiopathic or secondary to intraocular tumour, fibrous bands in diabetes or trauma. Fifty per cent of patients have the sensation of flashing lights or retinal spots before detachment. Painless loss of vision is characteristic, often with the description of a curtain being drawn over a part of the eye. Most detachments are visible on ophthalmoscopic examination as a grey forward-bulging area on the retina, but proper examination by an ophthalmologist is required to exclude the diagnosis. Prompt referral for treatment is required so that the detached segment may be secured in place.

Q181
a T b T c F d T e T

Acute angle closure glaucoma is a condition of middle to later life characterized by painful loss or reduction of vision. Blurring of vision or halo lights may precede the attack. The initial management includes instillation of pilocarpine drops 2–4% hourly and a stat dose of acetazolamide 500 mg followed by 250 mg 8-hourly. Urgent referral for ophthalmological opinion is required if the vision is to be saved.

Q182
a F b T c F d F e F

Acute iritis presents with an acutely painful red eye associated with photophobia and blurring of vision. The pupil is small and irregular. Talbot's test (increasing pain and pupillary constriction on convergence) is positive. Slit-lamp examination reveals white precipitates on the back of the cornea and pus in the anterior chamber (hypopyon). Treatment is with steroid drops to reduce inflammation and cyclopentolate 0.5–1.0% drops 6-hourly to dilate the pupil and therefore prevent adhesions between the lens and iris (synechiae). The condition should be managed by an ophthalmologist as regular slit lamp examination is required. Recurrence is common. As a general rule, steroid eye drops should not be prescribed in the A&E department.

Miscellaneous

Q183
a T b F c T d F e F

Children who have swallowed foreign bodies require X-ray studies to exclude aspiration or impaction in the oesophagus. The management of swallowed batteries is controversial: the type of battery must be identified and advice must be sought, as removal (before the battery disintegrates) may be appropriate. Aspirated foreign bodies usually require removal at bronchoscopy.

Q184
a T b T c T d T e T

Drowning is commonly associated with alcohol intoxication in young adults and is commonly associated with cervical spine injury. Cerebral oedema is a common sequela to near drowning, as is hypothermia. Haemolysis does not occur after sea-water drowning because of the high concentration of electrolytes in sea-water.

Q185
a F b T c F d T e T

The 'bends' are caused by nitrogen coming out of solution following decompression after a dive. Symptoms may appear up to 36 hours after the dive. Air travel should be avoided for 12 hours after the end of a dive.

Q186
a F b F c T d T e F

The standard pulse oximeter can only detect reduced and oxygenated haemoglobin and will therefore not detect carboxyhaemoglobin. Because of the shape of the oxygen dissociation curve, the pulse oximeter is effective at detecting desaturation, but cannot be used to indicate overly high levels of Pa_{O_2}. Skin colour and most nail varnishes have no effect on the reading.

Q187
a F b T c T d T e F

The management of anaphylaxis follows the basic pattern of any resuscitation; the airway is secured and high-flow oxygen administered. Adrenaline is given by the subcutaneous or IM route, except in severe or unresponsive anaphylaxis when the IV route may be used (1 ml aliquots of 1:10 000 adrenaline). Gaining IV access should not however delay administration of adrenaline. Hydrocortisone takes several hours to act and is therefore not a first-line drug. Wheeze is treated by nebulized β_2-agonist in the first instance. Aminophylline is a second-line drug.

Q188
a F b T c F d T e T

Decompression sickness results from nitrogen leaving solution in the blood and forming bubbles which are then transported within the circulation to different parts of the body to cause the syndrome known as the 'bends'. These are musculoskeletal pains around synovial joints which initially flit from joint to joint before becoming localized and increasingly painful. The commonest sites are the shoulder and knee. The 'chokes' comprise dyspnoea and chest pain (pneumothorax must be excluded). Vertigo and nausea are known as the 'staggers'. Other symptoms and signs include rashes, neurological symptoms (headache, behavioural disturbance, paraparesis, bladder and sphincter disturbances and unconsciousness) and circulatory effects, including hypertension. The treatment of choice is recompression.

Q189
a T b T c F d F e F

The incidence of drowning is highest in two age groups, toddlers and teenagers. Teenage males are common victims because of their risk-taking behaviour. A 'wet drowning' means that aspiration of water occurred during the immersion. Treatment is the same in salt- or fresh-water drowning. The most important phase of this treatment occurs before arrival at hospital, with effective management of the airway and ventilation. There is no evidence to support the use of prophylactic antibiotics or corticosteroids.

Q190
a T b T c F d F e F

Cooling down burns reduces the area and depth of the final burn by reducing the effect of heat transferred to the tissues. Care must be taken, however, with burns with a large area as cooling may make the patient hypothermic; in such situations a towel soaked in cold water may be used. Fluid loss is related to body weight and the surface area of the burn. Several formulae exist for calculating fluid requirements. Charts are available for estimating surface area of a burn: in adults the 'rule of nines' may be used. IV opiates are the analgesic of choice for burns, adequate analgesia reduces the adverse effects of the metabolic response to trauma. In general, escharotomy need only be performed in the A&E department for full thickness circumferential burns of the limbs causing circulatory embarrassment or of the chest causing respiratory embarrassment. Prophylactic antibiotics are not generally used for burns as they encourage the emergence of resistant strains – a major problem in burns units.

Q191
a T b F c F d T e T

Alternating current (e.g. the normal domestic supply) is more likely to produce ventricular fibrillation than is direct current. Lightning strike produces a massive direct current countershock which usually results in asystole, but only rarely results in skin damage. The current usually passes over the surface of the body ('flashover') causing either sudden cardiac death or burns as the water in wet clothing is vaporized. Direct current shock from other causes produces a small entrance and a much larger exit wound. Renal failure in electric shock results from myoglobinuria secondary to muscle breakdown. Bony injury from the victim being thrown by contact with an electrical source should always be excluded.

Q192
a F **b** T **c** T **d** T **e** T

Hydrofluoric acid is a colourless liquid used in the manufacturing industries and in the home as rust remover. Most burns occur on the hands or arm and are intensely painful. The fluoride ion can diffuse through the skin and cause systemic toxicity and death. Initial treatment should consist of lavage to decontaminate the wound. If the wound is still painful after lavage it indicates that there has been some penetration of the fluoride ion – 2.5% calcium gluconate gel should then be applied. The calcium conjugates with the fluoride ion to prevent any further systemic absorption.

Q193
a F **b** F **c** T **d** T **e** F

One millilitre of 1% solution of any drug contains 10 mg of that drug. Ten millilitres therefore contains 100 mg. The maximum safe dosage of plain lignocaine is 3–5 mg/kg. This increases to 7 mg/kg if adrenaline is added. Methaemoglobinaemia is a side-effect of the use of prilocaine.

Q194
a T **b** T **c** F **d** F **e** T

Children should receive a primary course of tetanus immunization consisting of three doses starting at 2 months with an interval of 1 month between each dose. A booster dose should be given prior to school entry and also before leaving school. A person who has completed a full course of tetanus vaccination within the last 10 years will not need any further prophylaxis. (A further dose of vaccine can be considered for a tetanus-prone wound if the risk of infection is felt to be very high.) Immunoglobulin should be given to the non-immunized patient with a tetanus-prone wound and a full course of vaccination should be commenced. The immunoglobulin is not necessary if the wound is clean and it is not contraindicated in those who are allergic to the vaccine.

Q195
a T b T c T d F e T

Silver sulphadiazine cream can be used for the prophylaxis and treatment of burn wounds. When used on the hand, application of a plastic bag allows early movement. Incised facial wounds may be left uncovered or treated with a non-stick film dressing.

Q196
a T b T c T d T e F

Entonox is a compressed gas consisting of 50% nitrous oxide and 50% oxygen. It is usually delivered through a patient-demand valve. It is therefore difficult to receive too much and does not cause any physiological changes of note. Cooling of the cylinder results in separation of liquid nitrous oxide. The possibility then exists of the patient receiving a hypoxic mixture of gases. This can be prevented by shaking the cylinder before use. Nitrous oxide diffuses into closed spaces faster than nitrogen can diffuse out. It is therefore contraindicated in patients with pneumothorax or the 'bends'.

Q197
a T b F c F d T e T

All wounds caused by a dog bite are dirty. It is said that the contamination caused by a dog bite is second in severity only to that of the human bite. The general principles of management are adequate wound cleaning and debridement, tetanus prophylaxis and antibiotic prophylaxis. Wounds should be left open and inspected regularly unless deep structures or bone or joint are involved, when debridement under general anaesthesia may be followed by primary closure. There is controversy over the choice of antibiotic. We use a simple agent initially (e.g. flucloxacillin or erythromycin 250–500 mg 6-hourly) and review the wound daily for the first few days, adding metronidazole if required. Others used a broad-spectrum agent such as co-amoxiclav (Augmentin) 375 mg 8-hourly. Significant bites should be X-rayed to exclude an underlying fracture or foreign body; osteomyelitis is uncommon.

Q198
a F b F c T d T e F

Burns involving the hand should be mobilized early to prevent
contracture and stiffness. This is best achieved by placing the hand in
a plastic bag and coating the hand in a water based cream (e.g.
Flamazine) to prevent it adhering to the bag. Blisters should not be
deroofed because the underlying exposed skin becomes infected. If a
blister is interfering with function (e.g. a blister on the hand) then it
may be aspirated under aseptic conditions. Silver sulphadiazine cream
should be avoided on the face as the silver can lead to a black
discoloration.

Q199
a T b T c T d T e T

Torticollis without underlying cause is common and is usually
noticed on waking. It can be caused by cervical disc prolapse, which
may be associated with upper limb paraesthesia, although weakness is
rare. Other causes of adult torticollis include neck trauma, ocular
disorders, vertebral infection and inflamed lymph nodes in the neck.

Q200
a T b T c T d F e F

Needlestick injuries are common and there is usually a local policy
which should be followed. Tetanus immunization should be offered to
those not covered. Seroconversion to HIV-positive status is extremely
rare worldwide after needlestick injury from needles used on
HIV-positive patients. Hepatitis B immunoglobulin should be offered
to staff whose titres are low; it is usually possible to measure titres
within the time scale for administering immunoglobulin (48 hours).

CASE HISTORIES

Case 1

A 31-year-old man presented complaining of severe low back pain and an ache in the right groin. He said this developed following a fall down a flight of stairs earlier that morning. He gave a complicated past history. As a child he had a perforated appendix and peritonitis. Ten years ago, he had been involved in a serious road traffic accident where he had been trapped in his vehicle. A tracheostomy had been performed, following which he had been extricated from the car. Further investigation, he said, had shown that he had a ruptured spleen and a fractured lumbar spine. He made a full recovery from his injuries. He mentioned that he is allergic to aspirin-like drugs.

On examination the following findings were noted:

- Tracheostomy scar and scars of the previous laparotomies and from two drain sites.
- Straight-leg-raising reduced to 20° on the right and 30° on the left. Hip flexion reduced in power on both sides.
- Decreased sensation to pinprick over the upper outer right thigh.
- Tenderness present over the second and third lumbar vertebrae. Rectal examination and perianal sensation were intact.
- Further examination was normal.

Questions

1 What is the differential diagnosis?
2 What investigations would you perform?

Case 2

A 24-year-old male was brought to the department after being resuscitated from a cardiac arrest at the university running track. The paramedic crew who attended the patient said that when they arrived, bystander cardiopulmonary resuscitation was taking place. They attached their monitor/defibrillator and found the patient to be in ventricular fibrillation. Following one shock at 200 J the patient's rhythm returned to sinus with an easily palpable pulse. The paramedics had then brought him straight to the department.

The patient's girlfriend who followed the ambulance to the hospital said that he had been previously well. However she mentioned that he had been complaining of feeling increasingly breathless over the past 2 weeks. She also said that his father had died from unknown causes when he was young.

On examination the following findings were noted:

- Patient conscious but confused in time and place.
- Pulse 56 beats/min sinus rhythm, normal character, blood pressure 125/75 mmHg.
- Apex beat felt as double impulse but undisplaced.
- Normal first and second heart sounds with late systolic murmur heard best at the apex.
- Lungs clinically clear.

Immediate investigations
- Portable (anteroposterior) chest X-ray appears normal.
- Twelve-lead ECG shows left ventricular hypertrophy and minor non-specific lateral ST segment changes.

Questions

1 What is the most likely diagnosis?
2 How would you confirm the diagnosis?
3 How would you manage this patient?

Case 3

A 24-year-old Negro student attended the department complaining of severe pain in his chest, upper back and extremities. He could not speak any English and no further history was possible.

On examination the following findings were noted:

- Patient appeared in severe pain, writhing on examination couch.
- Temperature 38.2°C.
- Chest clinically clear.
- Further examination normal.

Immediate investigations
- 12-lead ECG normal.
- Chest X-ray normal.
- Urinalysis: haematuria ++.

Questions

1 What diagnosis do you suspect?
2 How would you confirm this diagnosis?
3 What is your initial management of this patient?

Case 4

A young male aged 18 was brought into the department at 3 a.m. by two of his friends. He is agitated and confused. They said that they had been at a rave party when he had begun acting oddly. Then he collapsed to the floor and began shaking uncontrollably. After a minute this had stopped and he had gradually come around. They had brought him straight to the department in the back of their car. He had not had anything alcoholic to drink and as far as they knew he had not taken any drugs. No other history was available about the patient.

On examination the following findings were noted:

- Patient confused, disoriented in time, place and person.
- Generalized increase of muscle tone.
- Hot – temperature 40.6°C.
- No skin rash.
- Clinically dehydrated.
- Pulse 128 beats/min regular, poor volume, blood pressure 150/100 mmHg
- Pupils widely dilated.
- No focal neurological signs.

Questions

1 What is the most likely diagnosis?
2 How would you treat this young man?
3 Name two similar syndromes.

Case 5

A general practitioner rang the A&E department. He said that he had a 65-year-old diabetic woman in his surgery complaining of an acutely painful left eye. The patient could hardly see out of the eye, which had been watering heavily for 2 hours. She had vomited repeatedly whilst in the practice waiting room.

The GP had noted the following findings:

- Corrected vision right eye 6/6, left eye could see hand only.
- Left cornea cloudy.
- Left pupil fixed in mid-dilation and oval in shape.

Questions

1 What diagnosis do you suspect?
2 What other features would help you confirm the diagnosis?
3 What course of action would you recommend to the GP?

Case 6

A 43-year-old man was brought to the A&E department by an ambulance after being found collapsed in the street. The paramedics said that he smelt heavily of alcohol and that they had found an empty bottle of wine next to him.

On examination the following findings were noted:

- Unkempt.
- Temperature 36.2°C.
- Pulse 88 beats/min regular, good volume, blood pressure 146/84 mmHg.
- Respiratory rate 14 breaths/min.
- Vocalizing with incoherent sentences.
- 4 cm bleeding wound over occiput.

Immediate investigations
- BM 6.7 mmol/l.

Question

Discuss how you would assess and manage this patient.

Case 7

A 23-year-old man was brought to the A&E department at 7 a.m. by ambulance, accompanied by his parents. He had last been seen at 11 p.m. the previous night, when he returned from an evening out. His mother said that he had been complaining of a sore throat and had decided to go to bed early. At 6.30 a.m. his father had gone to wake him for work and found him unrousable, so called an ambulance. There was no past medical history of note.

On examination the following findings were noted:

- Temperature 38.4°C.
- Pulse 108 beats/min regular and thready, blood pressure 90/60 mmHg.
- Respiratory rate 24 breaths/min.
- Faint purpuric rash present over trunk.
- Glasgow Coma Score 3.

Investigations
- BM 3.2 mmol/l.

Question

Discuss how you would manage this patient.

Case 8

A 23-year-old known asthmatic was admitted to the A&E department at 4 a.m. with an acute exacerbation of her condition. No history was obtainable from the patient as she was too breathless to speak. Her father said that she had been wheezy most of the day and had commenced a course of oral prednisolone 40 mg daily the previous morning. She had been taking regular salbutamol inhalers and using her home nebulizer. She also used a steroid inhaler and took twice-daily slow-release aminophylline.

On examination the following findings were noted:

- Temperature 37.6°C.
- Pulse 148 beats/min regular, blood pressure 110/60 mmHg.
- Respiratory rate 40 breaths/min, sitting forward fighting for breath.
- Peripherally cyanosed.
- Chest clinically silent.

Investigations
- BM 4.4 mmol/l.
- Peak flow unrecordable.
- Blood gases on air
  Pao_2 6.6 kPa
  $Paco_2$ 7.8 kPa
  pH 7.24
  Base excess −9

Question

Discuss how you would manage this case.

Case 9

A 43-year-old man was admitted by ambulance to the A&E department. He had been found unconscious in his car with a hose pipe connected to the exhaust feeding into the window.
  On examination the following findings were noted:

- Temperature 36.2°C.
- Pulse 110 beats/min, blood pressure 128/78 mmHg.
- Respiratory rate 18 breaths/min.
- Glasgow Coma Score 3.

Investigations
- BM 5.2 mmol/l.
- Blood gases on air
  Pao_2 9.6 kPa.
  $Paco_2$ 4.8 kPa.
  pH 7.22
  Base excess −14
- Full blood count (FBC): Hb 15.2 g/dl, White cell count (WCC) 15.2 $\times 10^9$/l, platelets 344 $\times 10^9$/l
- Urea and electrolytes (U + Es): Na^+ 136 mmol/l, K^+ 2.8 mmol/l, urea 5.8 mmol/l.
- Carboxyhaemoglobin (COHb) level 8%.

Question

Discuss how you would manage this patient.

Case 10

A 56-year-old man presented to the department with a 1-hour history of crushing central chest pain radiating down the left arm. He had vomited once. The pain had developed whilst at a meeting at work. In the past he had been well, apart from occasional pain from a duodenal ulcer. He smoked 30 cigarettes a day. His father had died of a heart attack at the age of 54. The only medication that the man took regularly was ranitidine 300 mg at night. He admitted to the occasional use of cocaine.

On examination the following findings were noted:

- Patient in pain, sweaty and clammy.
- Pulse 76 beats/min regular, blood pressure 138/88 mmHg.
- Cardiac examination normal.
- Respiratory rate 16 breaths/min.
- Chest clear.

Investigations
- BM 4.8 mmol/l.
- Portable chest X-ray normal.
- 12-lead ECG: rate 80 bpm, sinus rhythm. Hyperacute changes of an anterolateral myocardial infarction.

Question

Discuss how you would manage this case.

Case 11

A 60-year-old man presented to the A&E department with a history of sudden painless loss of vision in the right eye. This had developed 2 hours previously. The man suffered with hypertension and angina. He was short-sighted but had no other history of eye problems. His medication was aspirin 150 mg daily, a slow-release oral nitrate and GTN spray when necessary.

On examination the following findings were noted:

- Apyrexial.
- Pulse 80 beats/min regular, blood pressure 160/90 mmHg.
- No cardiac murmurs, no bruits heard in neck.

- Respiratory rate 12 breaths/min, chest clear.
- Visual acuity in the right eye is to fingers only, in the left eye 6/18.
- Fundoscopy shows a 'stormy sunset' appearance with hyperaemia, engorged veins and haemorrhages alongside the veins.

Investigations
- BM stick: 5.4 mmol/l.
- FBC: Hb 14.6 g/dl, WCC 8.4 $\times 10^9$/l, platelets 378 $\times 10^9$/l.
- ESR: 16.

Questions

1 What is the diagnosis?
2 How would you manage this patient?

Case 12.

A 10-year-old boy was brought to the department because of a limp. This had been noticed at school and he had been sent home. The boy said that his left thigh was painful. Three days ago he had played a game of football for his school but he could not remember any injury. His mother mentioned that he had suffered with a cold about 10 days ago but this had resolved. There was no past history or family history of hip problems.

On examination these were the findings:

- Pyrexial, temperature 37.9°C.
- Enlarged tonsils.
- Chest clear.
- Mild spasm in muscles of left hip.
- Abduction and internal rotation limited when compared with right hip.
- Left knee non-tender with full range of movement.

Questions

1 What is your differential diagnosis?
2 What investigations will you arrange?

Case 13.

A 25-year-old woman came to the department complaining of shortness of breath and fast regular palpitations. She said that she had noticed the fast heart rate whilst sitting at her computer terminal at work. Shortly afterwards she became short of breath.

The previous week she said she had visited her GP with a similar feeling of breathlessness. He had told her that she was hyperventilating and advised her to breathe into a paper bag if she ever developed similar symptoms. She had tried that this morning but it had not helped. Six months previously she had been admitted with a paracetamol overdose after an argument with her fiancé.

Her mother was asthmatic but there was no other family history of illness. She lived with her fiancé and worked as a keyboard operator for a mail-order company. The only regular medication that she took was the combined oral contraceptive pill. She was a non-smoker and drank about eight units of alcohol a week.

On examination the findings were:

- Anxious lady, hyperventilating with rapid shallow breaths into a paper bag.
- Well-hydrated.
- Temperature 37.5°C.
- Good peripheral colour and not cyanosed.
- Pulse 120 beats/min regular, good volume, blood pressure 140/90 mmHg.
- Heart sounds normal, no murmurs.
- Good air entry to both lungs, no wheeze heard.
- Further examination normal.

The following investigations had been performed:

- ECG: Sinus tachycardia, rate 120 bpm, no other abnormalities.
- Chest X-ray: Normal

Questions

1 What is your differential diagnosis?
2 What other investigations would you like to order?

Case 14

An 18-month-old girl was brought to the department with a painful left thumb. Her mother remembered that whilst driving her car 2 days previously, she had braked sharply to avoid an accident. Her

118

daughter, who was restrained in a baby seat in the back of the vehicle, had been thrown forward in her restraining straps. Later that evening the girl had started rubbing her left thumb and complained that her hand was sore. The woman had taken her daughter to her GP who had sent her to the A&E department for an X-ray.

On examination the following findings were noted:

- Happy 18-month-old baby.
- No obvious swelling or deformity of thumb.
- No bony tenderness.
- Full range of flexion of thumb interphalangeal joint.
- Extension decreased by 40° at thumb interphalangeal joint.

Investigation
- X-ray of thumb and metacarpal: no fracture or dislocation seen.

Questions

1 What is the likely diagnosis?
2 How would you treat this patient?

Case 15

A radio-call was received in the department from an ambulance bringing in a cardiac arrest. A man in his 50s had been found floating unconscious in his swimming pool by his wife when she had returned from visiting a friend. The cardiac arrest team was assembled when the patient arrived.

As the patient was transferred to the resuscitation trolley the paramedic informed the team that when they arrived the patient was not breathing and had no pulse. They had intubated, started cardiac massage and then brought him straight to the hospital.

On initial assessment the following findings are noted:

- Patient intubated and tube tied in place.
- Good air entry to both lungs using self-inflating bag with oxygen reservoir.
- No spontaneous pulse. Good pulse with cardiac massage.
- Pupils bilaterally fixed and dilated.

As the initial assessment was taking place these investigations were performed:

- ECG monitor: fine ventricular fibrillation.
- BM stick: 8.3 mmol/l.
- Rectal temperature 27°C.

Questions

1 What important step in the initial assessment of the patient has been omitted?
2 How would you manage this patient?

Case 16

A young mother brought her $2\frac{1}{2}$-year-old boy to the department saying that he had swallowed a battery. This was a button-type cell that had fallen out of an electric toy that a friend had brought back from holiday in Singapore. Unfortunately it was not possible to determine the exact type of battery. He had swallowed it about 3 hours before the presentation in A&E and had been well since.
   On clinical examination no abnormal findings were noted.

Investigations
- X-ray of chest and upper abdomen – button battery visible apparently lying in the fundus of the stomach.

Questions

1 How would you manage this patient?
2 Would your management have differed if the battery was in the small bowel?
3 What type of button batteries are associated with a high risk of danger?

Case 17

A 78-year-old woman was brought to the department after falling whilst out collecting her shopping. She said that she had felt suddenly light-headed and had fallen to the ground. She had not been unconscious at any time but had been too weak to stand up. She mentioned that she had been passing urine more frequently over the past 2 days but had not noticed any dysuria.

She was now complaining of an aching pain in her right hip. Apart from a broken right wrist 3 years previously, she had been remarkably fit. Her husband had died the previous year and she lived alone in their detached bungalow. Both of her children had emigrated and her only other family was an elder sister who was resident in a nursing home. She was still quite active, attending her local bowls club twice a week, and did not receive any social service support. Her GP had recently started her on a water tablet because of her swollen ankles. She could not remember the exact name of the medication. She also took nitrazepam 10 mg at night.

On examination the following findings were noted:

- Pleasant woman who appeared in pain.
- Mucous membranes pink.
- Temperature 37.8°C.
- Pulse 140 beats/min irregularly irregular.
- Blood pressure 150/95 mmHg sitting.
- Jugular venous pressure raised 4 cm.
- Heart sounds normal, no murmurs heard.
- Bilateral fine end-inspiratory crepitations heard in chest.
- Abdominal examination normal.
- Early bruising apparent over left hip.
- Legs of equal length.
- Movement of left hip painful.
- Neurological examination normal.

Questions

1 What is your differential diagnosis?
2 What investigations would you arrange?
3 Outline the principles of managing the elderly patient presenting with a history of collapse.

Case 18

A young woman rushed into the department in an agitated state. The triage nurse took the woman to a cubicle and ascertained that she was suffering with a vaginal bleed. On further questioning by the A&E doctor the woman said that she was 10 weeks pregnant. Her pregnancy had been confirmed by a test at her GP's surgery. She was upset because she had suffered two previous miscarriages and was worrried this might happen again. She was otherwise fit and well. Her periods had been regular before the pregnancy and there was no other relevant gynaecological history.

On examination the following findings were noted:

- Upset woman.
- Mucous membranes pink.
- Apyrexial.
- Pulse 88 beats/min regular, good volume, blood pressure 110/75 mmHg.
- Cardiovascular and respiratory systems normal.
- Abdomen – uterus not palpable; minimally tender in suprapubic region.
- Speculum – small amount of blood in vagina, os healthy-looking and closed.
- Vaginal examination – no tenderness elicited, no cervical excitation.

Investigation
- Urinary pregnancy test positive.

Questions

1 What is the likely diagnosis?
2 How would you manage this patient?

Case 19

A 25-year-old man attended the department complaining of intermittent headaches. He said these had developed after a head injury 1 week previously. He had been playing football when he had clashed heads with another player. Although he had not been knocked out, he had been dizzy for 30 minutes and could not complete the game. He said he had gone to the local A&E department at the time but they had said he had not suffered any serious injury and he could go home. The following morning he had awoken with a headache. He said it was all over his head. It was eased by paracetamol but had usually recurred by the end of the day. On further questioning the patient mentioned that he also felt light-headed and lethargic and was having difficulty concentrating at work.

On examination the following findings were noted:

- Patient appears unhappy.
- Apyrexial.
- Pulse 64 beats/min regular, blood pressure 110/80 mmHg.
- Pupils equal and react to light and accommodate.
- Fundoscopy normal.
- Cranial nerves grossly intact.
- No focal neurological deficit.
- Rest of examination normal.

Questions

1 What is the likely diagnosis?
2 How would you treat this patient?
3 What symptoms and signs would encourage you to arrange a cranial CT in a patient with a headache?

Case 20

A young man was brought into the resuscitation room by an ambulance paramedic crew. They said that the patient, a 25-year-old man, lost control of his motorbike whilst taking a corner too fast in wet conditions. They found him some 30 metres from the motorbike lying against a tree. The patient was conscious when the paramedics arrived. They had immobilized his neck in a rigid collar with sandbags and tape on a full-length spinal board. High-concentration oxygen using a mask with a reservoir bag had been administered and the paramedics had inserted a large-bore cannula and started a colloid drip. They said he had become increasingly distressed during the journey to the hospital, complaining of pain over the right side of the chest.

On initial assessment in A&E the following findings were noted:

- Patient unconscious, making grunting noises. After simple airway manoeuvres were applied the airway became unobstructed.
- Trachea deviated to the left.
- Neck veins engorged.
- Chest expansion unequal and decreased on the right.
- Chest hyper-resonant on the right.
- Air entry decreased on the right.

Questions

1 What are the simple ways with which an airway can be maintained
  without having to resort to endotracheal intubation or a surgical
  airway?
2 What diagnosis do you suspect and how would you treat this
  condition?
3 What will be your next stage in the management of this patient?

ANSWERS TO CASE HISTORY QUESTIONS

Case 1

1 Nerve root compression at L2/L3 disc level.
Meralgia paraesthetica.
Münchausen's syndrome.
2 Attempt to confirm past history.
X-ray of lumbar spine.
Further imaging of lumbar spine.
Perform diagnostic local block of lateral cutaneous nerve of thigh.

This patient has suffered a fall and now has tenderness in the region of his second and third lumbar vertebrae, together with paraesthesiae of the upper outer thigh and weakness of hip flexion. This could all suggest compression of the second lumbar nerve root as it exits between the lumbar vertebrae, due to a compression fracture. A second possibility is meralgia paraesthetica, a condition caused by compression of the lateral cutaneous nerve of the thigh as it passes under the inguinal ligament medial to the anterior superior iliac spine. This is not usually a result of trauma but may be the first sign of a metastatic lesion affecting the second and third lumbar nerve root.

The unusual history (a tracheostomy at the scene of an accident is not a frequent occurrence) and the plethora of scars present on the patient should alert the clinician to the possibility of Münchausen's syndrome, or chronic factitious disorder, which was the correct diagnosis.

The first investigation should be to try and corroborate the history. Many A&E departments carry special lists of patients with Münchausen's syndrome so neighbouring units should be contacted. Although patients may not give a correct name, they do usually give other correct details, such as a date of birth or a GP who can provide further avenues for enquiries.

If the past history proves to be correct, then the other diagnoses should be considered. X-rays of the lumbar spine should be performed because of the history of trauma to exclude a fracture in the region of L2 or L3 and also to exclude any other bony pathology in this region. If an abnormality is discovered and the diagnosis of nerve root compression is suspected then further imaging techniques may be needed. Nuclear magnetic resonance provides the best results in this area. If the motor function of L2 is normal then meralgia paraesthetica should be considered. Injection of local anaesthetic into the region of the lateral cutaneous nerve of the thigh as it exits under the inguinal ligament with subsequent prompt resolution of the symptoms would confirm the diagnosis.

Münchausen's syndrome was first described in 1951 by Asher and named after an 18th-century nobleman who was famed for his story-telling. Patients often present with elaborate and convincing medical histories and may have florid signs. The whole clinical presentation can be seen as an attempted deception of the medical staff. Recent work has suggested that it is not as uncommon as previously suspected. Some cases may have underlying brain damage. It is a notoriously difficult condition to treat and can result in great financial and emotional stress on the medical system. Powell and Boast suggest that many of these patients should fall under the provision of the Mental Health Act, in which case they would be able to be offered care appropriate to their disorder. In the A&E department of today the patient should be offered psychiatric referral and counselling, though many will refuse.

References

Lawrie SM, Goodwin G, Masterson G (1993) Münchausen's syndrome and organic brain disorder. *Br. J. Psychiatry* **162**: 545–549

Leland DG (1993) Münchausen's syndrome: a brief review. *S.D.J.Med* **46**: 109–112

Powell L, Boast L (1993) The million dollar man. Resource implications for chronic Münchausen's syndrome. *Br. J. Psychiatry* **162**: 253–256

Case 2

1 Hypertrophic obstructive cardiomyopathy (HOCM).
2 Echocardiography.
3 Give the patient oxygen, insert a cannula and institute cardiac monitoring. Refer to physicians to arrange admission, further investigations and treatment.

HOCM is characterized by hypertrophy of the left and occasionally the right ventricles. Inheritance is usually autosomal dominant and the male-to-female ratio is 1:1. This patient's father may have suffered with the same condition. HOCM presents from the neonatal period to old age, most commonly in the second decade, with shortness of breath precipitated by exercise. Arrhythmias are common and may be ventricular or supraventricular. The double apex impulse is due to a palpable atrial filling thrust trying to overcome the obstruction caused by the hypertrophic muscle. The late systolic murmur is caused by mitral incompetence secondary to distortion of the mitral valve ring.

In symptomatic patients, a normal ECG is rare. Abnormalities include left (and right) ventricular hypertrophy and ST segment and T-wave abnormalities. Left bundle branch block may occur.

The investigation of choice is the M-mode echocardiogram. The findings characteristic of HOCM are a greatly thickened septum, systolic anterior motion of the the aortic valve and early closure of the aortic valve cusps. Occasionally it may be necessary to perform left ventricular angiography to confirm the diagnosis.

Treatment should be aimed at reducing the symptoms and also at reducing the risk of fatal ventricular arrhythmias. β-Blockers are usually used and improve symptoms but have little effect on arrhythmias. If frequent ventricular arrhythmias are apparent on ambulatory electrocardiography then therapy with amiodarone should be considered. If patients do not respond to medical treatment, surgery can be performed to resect the septal hypertophy but results are poor.

Case 3

1 Vaso-occlusive crisis in patient with sickle cell anaemia.
2 Request an interpreter so that the full history can be obtained. Full blood count and reticulocyte count. Sickledex. Look at peripheral blood smear for sickled cells.
3 Give patient oxygen, intravenous fluids and intravenous pain relief. Refer to medical team for admission and further investigation.

The most likely diagnosis in this patient is an acute vaso-occlusive crisis in a patient with sickle-cell anaemia. Most of these patients will know the cause of their pain so the past history should be ascertained as soon as possible. A positive Sickledex and examination of the peripheral blood for sickled red cells may also indicate the diagnosis. However there is no test immediately available that can confirm if the patient is in a crisis. Some patients may in fact be analgesic abusers with coincidental sickle cell disease.

Pain results from infarction secondary to vaso-occlusion and may occur in the liver, spleen, lungs, brain and most commonly bone. Sickle-cell crises are precipitated by hypoxia, dehydration, infection, acidosis or exposure to cold temperatures. An FBC will demonstrate a haemoglobin of 6–8 g/dl with a reticulocyte count of 10–20%. The haemoglobin remains stable during a pain crisis unless aplasia, haemolysis or sequestration occurs. Haemolysis and aplasia may be secondary to infection, so blood cultures and a full infection screen should be performed. Blood gases should be checked to look for hypoxia. Other investigations will depend on the symptoms with which the patient has presented. In this case the haematuria was due to renal papillary necrosis.

The emergency treatment of these patients should commence with additional oxygen and intravenous fluids. Pain relief should be given with intravenous opiates. However, the possibility of analgesic abuse should also be borne in mind. Most hospitals that see large numbers of these patients will have a protocol for giving adequate pain relief and will have records of known analgesic abusers. The patient should be re-examined after 30 minutes and further pain relief given if necessary. He should be referred to the inpatient medical team for further assessment of the cause and treatment of the crisis.

Long-term complications of sickle cell disease include susceptibility to infection, particularly meningitis and osteomyelitis, gallstones, ischaemic leg ulcers, aseptic necrosis of bone, cardiovascular disease, chronic renal disease and blindness due to retinal detachment or proliferative retinopathy.

Case 4

1 Hyperthermic syndrome as an adverse reaction to use of Ecstasy.
2 Stabilize airway, breathing and circulation.
   Paralyse and ventilate the patient.
   Administer dantrolene.
3 Malignant hyperpyrexia associated with anaesthetic agents.
   Malignant neuroleptic syndrome.

The clinical features of euphoria, restlessness, talkativeness, tachycardia, sweating, tachypnoea, tremor and dilated pupils suggest stimulant abuse. This patient also has a high temperature. The diagnosis of hyperthermic syndrome secondary to ingestion of Ecstasy should be suspected.

Ecstasy and E are street names for the drug 3,4-methylenedioxymethamphetamine (MDMA). This is a 'designer' drug that is currently popular with the rave culture in the UK. Although perceived to be safe, when taken in a hot environment with a low fluid intake and accompanying much physical activity, a heatstroke-like illness can result. Other side effects of MDMA ingestion include cardiac arrhythmias, coma and psychiatric disturbances.

Urgent treatment must be instituted for this patient. There have been no reported survivors when the patient's temperature has risen above 42°C. Supportive care of the patient's airway, breathing and circulation should be commenced. Cooling measures should then be instituted. The most effective intervention is to paralyse and ventilate the patient. This stops muscular movement and so decreases thermogenesis. In addition dantrolene should be given. This works by uncoupling the excitation–contraction process at the sarcoplasmic reticulum, thus blocking the thermogenic cycle. External cooling with ice packs or cooling blankets and internal cooling with cold saline infusions or cooled peritoneal or pleural lavage should also be commenced. When the patient has been intubated the opportunity can also be taken to wash the stomach out and install activated charcoal to minimize absorption of the drug.

Routine investigations should include FBC, blood gases, coagulation profile (disseminated intravascular coagulation is a complication), urea and electrolytes (hyponatraemia is frequently reported), liver function tests and cross-match. Blood, urine and gastric aspirates should be sent for drug screening. The patient will need to be monitored on the intensive care unit.

There are several closely related conditions that may present to the A&E department. Malignant hyperpyrexia is an inherited abnormality of skeletal muscle cells in which an exposure to anaesthetic drugs such as halothane or suxamethonium may precipitate a rapid rise in body temperature. Malignant neuroleptic syndrome is associated with the use of neuroleptic drugs such as the phenothiazines. Presentation tends to be less acute. There may be quite severe rhabdomyolysis with consequent renal failure. Dantrolene can be used if severe hyperpyrexia develops with either of these conditions.

References

Henry JA, Jeffreys KJ, Dawling S (1992) Toxicity and deaths from 3,4-methylenedioxy-methamphetamine ('ecstasy'). *Lancet* **340:** 384–387
O'Connor B (1994). Hazards associated with the recreational drug 'ecstasy'. *Br. J. Hosp. Med.* **52:** 507–514

Case 5

1 Acute angle closure glaucoma.
2 Globe appears dusky red.
Intraocular pressure raised on finger tonometry.
3 Send patient to nearest centre where on-call ophthalmological expertise is available.

The patient has acute angle closure glaucoma. She may have experienced painful premonitory attacks. Other clinical features of an attack of acute angle glaucoma include an intense dusky redness of the globe and dimness of the red reflex due to corneal clouding. The eye will feel rock hard on 'finger' tonometry and the anterior chamber, if visible, will be shallow.

Acute angle closure glaucoma is more common in high hypermetropes because of the shallow anterior chamber (*remember* – the spectacles of hypermetropic people magnify anything read through them).

The patient should be referred to the nearest A&E department at which ophthalmological expertise is available. A topical miotic (e.g. pilocarpine 4%) should be given every 5 minutes for five instillations from arrival and then 6-hourly. This will constrict the pupil, drawing the iris from the anterior chamber. Intravenous acetazolamide is given to reduce aqueous secretion and analgesia will be required. The other eye should receive prophylactic pilocarpine.

Case 6

The management of the drunk head injury is one of the more difficult areas of A&E medicine. These patients usually present at night when the least experienced doctor is available to manage them, they arouse little sympathy from nursing or medical staff and are difficult to assess. There are many accounts of the 'drunk' who died due to a missed intracranial bleed. The goal in managing drunken patients with a head injury is therefore to exclude significant intracranial pathology, to monitor them to ensure that their condition does not deteriorate and to ensure that there is no secondary pathology.

The initial assessment should include inspection of the airway to make sure it is clear and immobilization of the cervical spine if neck injury is thought likely. Ventilation and haemodynamic status should next be assessed. A pressure bandage should be applied to the scalp wound to prevent further haemorrhage and circulatory deterioration whilst the primary survey is completed. In this case no other injuries were found and the patient was haemodynamically stable. A more detailed assessment of his neurological condition should then be performed. In this case this revealed a GCS of 11 (verbal = 4, eye = 2, motor = 5), indicating a significant decrease in conscious level (a GCS of 8 or less indicates coma). It should never be assumed that a depressed GCS is secondary to alcohol or other drug intoxication. However as the pupillary reactions were normal and no focal neurological deficit was detectable, it would be reasonable to monitor this patient regularly rather than to proceed to CT scan.

There is no consensus view on how frequently neurological observations should be taken on the drunken head injury in the A&E department. In the early stages where change, if it is to occur, is likely to happen, observations should be frequent – every 15 minutes. It is usual to reduce this to hourly observations if the patient remains stable.

A depressed skull fracture should also be excluded in this patient. The cranial wound must be carefully inspected and palpated for a depressed fragment before the injury is sutured. If the history was strongly suggestive of a depressed fracture, skull X-rays should be taken. In the absence of this history radiographs are not mandatory if the patient is to be admitted. Furthermore they may be very difficult to achieve if the patient is in an agitated state. However, if the patient's GCS improves and he wishes to self-discharge, skull X-rays should be taken. The risk of an intracranial haematoma in a fully conscious patient rises from 1:1000 if there is no fracture to 1:30 with a fracture.

A blood alcohol measurement can also be of diagnostic help with these patients. If the level is <44 mmol/l then alcohol is very unlikely to be the cause of the coma. Alcohol meters and diagnostic sticks that can measure saliva alcohol are alternatives that are available in some departments.

Although it is generally taught that a drunken head injury should not be kept in the A&E department, it is our experience that these patients are rarely admitted unless there is an observation ward adjacent to the department. This patient's condition improved whilst he waited on a trolley in the department over the next 6 hours and he was discharged in the morning.

Case 7

The initial management, as with any emergency, should be rapidly to assess airway, breathing and circulation. This patient is clinically shocked and has the features of meningococcal meningitis. The purpuric rash indicates the presence of septicaemia. A large-bore cannula should be inserted and blood taken for culture. Benzylpenicillin 3 g IV stat should be given. Treatment should not be delayed to await the result of a lumbar puncture as death may ensue rapidly. IV fluids should be commenced to aim to restore the blood pressure.

A full clinical examination should now be performed to exclude any other conditions. The fundi should be examined for papilloedema, which will only be seen in late cases where intracranial pressure is very raised. Blood should be taken for FBC, electrolytes and glucose. A clotting screen is necessary to look for evidence of disseminated intravascular coagulation. Blood gases should be measured to assess oxygenation and acid–base status.

Lumbar puncture should be performed in the absence of papilloedema to confirm the diagnosis. Neither fundoscopy nor cranial CT can ensure with total certainty that the lumbar puncture will be safe. CT scan is not mandatory if the diagnosis is certain but should be performed if a cerebral abscess remains a possibility. The patient should be admitted to the intensive therapy unit and receive benzylpenicillin 3 g 4-hourly, unless microbiological tests indicate otherwise.

This is a notifiable disease, so the local Public Health Laboratory must be informed. Attempts should be made to trace any recent contacts of the patient. They should be offered rifampicin or ciprofloxacin to prevent possible development of the disease.

The most important principle in the management of suspected meningococcal meningitis is the early administration of high-dose benzylpenicillin. Delays in confirming the diagnosis or in performing microbiological tests have proved fatal. In the pre-hospital situation IM benzylpenicillin may be given. The use of IV dexamethasone has been shown to reduce mortality and morbidity in children with meningococcal meningitis/septicaemia if the dexamethasone is given with or shortly after the first dose of benzylpenicillin.

Case 8

This patient is suffering a life-threatening attack of asthma. The clinical indices all indicate a severe attack (British Thoracic Society (BTS) guidelines: pulse ≥ 125 beats/min, respirations ≥ 25 breaths/min, peak flow < 33% predicted, inability to speak and a silent chest are all indicators of severe/life-threatening asthma). In addition the blood gases indicate respiratory failure with acidosis

(BTS criteria for respiratory failure Pa_{O_2} <8 kPa and/or Pa_{CO_2} >6 kPa). This patient requires immediate intubation and ventilation.

When the patient's airway has been secured attention can be aimed at reducing bronchospasm. Nebulized salbutamol should be added to the inspiratory oxygen. IV infusion of salbutamol (5 µg/min) may also be tried. The volatile anaesthetic agents such as halothane are potent bronchodilators and can be very useful in this situation. Intravenous theophyllines should be avoided until theophylline levels can be determined. At that point an aminophylline infusion can be commenced. FBC and electrolytes should be measured and the blood gases repeated. A chest X-ray should be performed to exclude an iatrogenic pneumothorax which may have developed because of the high inflation pressures necessary with these patients. Transfer to the intensive care unit should be arranged as soon as possible.

Reference

British Thoracic Society guidelines for management of asthma (1993) Chart 6: asthma in accident and emergency departments. *Thorax* **48**: S23.

Case 9

The optimal treatment of carbon monoxide (CO) poisoning is controversial. After assessment and management of the airway, high-flow oxygen (aim for 100% with a rebreathing bag) should be administered. If respiration is adequate circulation should be assessed. Cardiac monitoring should be instituted and a 12-lead ECG requested because of the risk of myocardial ischaemia with CO poisoning. Blood should be sent for electrolyte estimation and cardiac enzymes. A chest X-ray should be taken to look for evidence of aspiration . A CO level may be performed. The normal range for COHb is <5% in a non-smoker, <10% in a smoker. The COHb is of little value itself unless the duration of exposure is known, the time since exposure and how much oxygen was given in that time. Similarly, pulse oximeter readings are unreliable because the standard oximeter does not detect COHb. The finding of a near normal Pa_{O_2} is common and should not affect the decision to give 100% oxygen. The underlying problem is utilization of oxygen within the cells, not the supply of oxygen.

The respiratory enzymes have half-lives in combination with CO of up to 48 hours (compared with 280 minutes for COHb). The COHb level may therefore be misleading. The common findings in

CO poisoning are a metabolic acidosis (which should not be treated aggressively with bicarbonate), hypokalaemia and a leukocytosis. Rhabdomyolysis is a later feature and leads to enormously raised creatine phosphokinase, following which renal failure may ensue.

Indications for transfer to a hyperbaric chamber include neurological symptoms (even if they occur several days after exposure), cardiac failure, irritability, personality changes and headache. As CO combined with respiratory enzymes has a long half-life, treatment may be beneficial even several days after exposure. The patient should be discussed with a physician at the hyperbaric unit before being transferred.

This patient will require intubation and ventilation for safe transfer. Propofol and atracurium are the drugs of choice. Midazolam and fentanyl are best avoided as the patient will need neurological assessment on arrival at the hyperbaric unit.

Case 10

After a rapid assessment of airway, breathing and cardiac output, oxygen should be administered by facemask at 4 l/min (there is no evidence that supplemental oxygen improves the outcome from myocardial infarction). Venous access should then be obtained using a peripheral cannula and blood taken for FBC, urea and electrolytes, glucose and cardiac enzymes. Soluble aspirin (in the absence of contraindications) 300 mg should be given. Pain relief can be achieved by giving a titrated dose of diamorphine 2.5–5 mg IV together with metoclopramide 10 mg IV as an antiemetic (prochlorperazine is not licensed for intravenous use). A brief clinical examination should be carried out, looking for evidence of murmurs and heart failure. A chest X-ray should not be allowed to delay further management. It may be deferred until the patient is admitted to the coronary care unit. This man is a prime candidate for early thrombolysis. In the absence of any contraindication streptokinase should be administered as an infusion. This may be performed in the A&E department or on the coronary care unit, but should be achieved within the current recognized standard of a 'door-to-needle' time of less than 30 minutes.

The combination of IV thrombolysis (any of the three available agents) and oral soluble aspirin reduces the mortality from myocardial infarction by 25%. Thrombolysis and aspirin contribute approximately equal proportions to the survival.

Case 11

1 Central retinal vein occlusion.
2 Refer to ophthalmologist.
  Treat underlying cause.

The differential diagnosis of painless loss of vision includes amaurosis fugax, ischaemic optic neuropathy, central retinal vein occlusion, central retinal artery occlusion, vitreous haemorrhage and retinal detachment.

The fundoscopic appearances in this patient are characteristic of central retinal vein occlusion. This occurs most commonly in the elderly; the incidence rises with increasing age. Predisposing factors include hypertension, atherosclerosis, chronic simple glaucoma and polycythaemia.

There is no specific treatment for this condition. Underlying causes such as hypertension, polycythaemia and chronic simple glaucoma should be identified and treated to reduce the possibility of a contralateral occurrence.

The outcome is variable. Improvement may occur for up to 1 year, particularly in peripheral vision. New vessel formation can predispose to secondary glaucoma (15% of cases) and intraocular haemorrhage.

Case 12

1 Transient synovitis of the hip.
  Slipped upper femoral epiphysis.
  Perthes' diease.
  Septic arthritis.
  Bony injury.
2 FBC, ESR and blood cultures.
  X-ray of both hips.
  Ultrasound of hip with aspiration if effusion detected.

The child with a painful hip is a common cause of diagnostic difficulties in the A&E department. Septic arthritis is the most important condition to exclude. A normal FBC and ESR make the diagnosis unlikely. Ultrasound of the hip should also be performed to look for an effusion. If fluid is present it can be aspirated under ultrasound guidance and sent for microscopy and culture.

Slipped upper femoral epiphysis affects children between the ages of 10 and 16. It is three times more common in males than females and the children tend to be obese. They present with a limp and pain in the groin, thigh or knee. Diagnosis is made by anteroposterior and lateral X-ray.

Perthes disease is an osteochondritis of the femoral head and can present with a similar picture. It usually affects children between the ages of 4 and 10 and is again more common in boys. The diagnosis is made on X-ray appearances. However, in the first stages of the disease the X-rays may appear normal.

Other causes of a painful hip in this age group include trauma and, if the patient has symptoms in other joints, juvenile rheumatoid arthritis.

If the investigations are normal then the diagnosis of exclusion is transient synovitis or 'irritable hip'. This condition, first described by Lovett and Morse in 1892, is characterized by pain felt in the hip and knee which often develops after a recent upper respiratory tract infection. It resolves spontaneously with bedrest but may recur. Follow-up should be arranged at 2–3 months to ensure that the symptoms are not the first indication of Perthes disease.

The FBC, ESR and X-rays of this patient were normal. An ultrasound of the hip showed a small effusion which was aspirated. The aspirate was clear and sterile. He was admitted under the orthopaedic team for bedrest and his condition settled over the next 2 days. A diagnosis of irritable hip was made. The patient was completely symptom-free at his 3-month review.

Case 13

1 Pulmonary embolism.
  Hyperventilation syndrome.
  Diabetic ketoacidosis.
  Aspirin overdose.
2 Urine for glucose and ketones.
  Arterial blood gases.
  Chest X-ray.
  Paracetamol and salicylate levels.

A young woman presenting with a rapid respiratory rate can all too easily be dismissed as suffering with hyperventilation syndrome and the true diagnosis missed. This woman has also noticed a fast heart rate. The combination of dyspnoea with tachycardia should make one think of the diagnosis of pulmonary embolism. Other causes of dyspnoea, such as pneumothorax, asthma and left ventricular failure, are unlikely because of the history and clinical signs.

A further diagnostic group of illnesses that should be considered are the causes of a metabolic acidosis. The respiratory rate would then be fast to try and compensate for the tissue acidosis. The most likely cause for a metabolic acidosis is diabetic ketoacidosis. Other possibilities are an aspirin overdose, which would also cause hyperventilation by direct respiratory stimulation, ingestion of methanol, renal failure and lactic acidosis.

Only when all of these diagnoses can be excluded should the hyperventilation syndrome be considered.

Investigations should be aimed at excluding these conditions. A urine sample should be dipsticked to look for the glucose and ketones of diabetic ketoacidosis. A chest X-ray should be taken if intrinsic lung disease is suspected and may also show oligaemic lung fields in the case of pulmonary embolism. Blood should be taken for electrolytes and paracetamol and salicylate levels if renal disease or overdose is suspected. Probably the most useful investigation is arterial blood gases which will show if the patient is hypoxic and reveal her acid–base status. The blood gases of this woman were as follows.

Blood gases taken on room air:

- Po_2: 11.1 kPa.
- Pco_2: 2.9 kPa.
- pH: 7.35.
- Base excess: −10.

The patient has a normal Po_2 according to the standard ranges. However, a patient with this degree of hyperventilation should have a high or high-normal Po_2. There is therefore some hypoxia compensated by the hyperventilation. The rest of the gases show a metabolic acidosis with partial respiratory compensation. These gases are highly indicative of the diagnosis of pulmonary embolism. The woman was heparinized immediately and a ventilation/perfusion scan performed that afternoon. Several mismatched defects were demonstrated consistent with a diagnosis of multiple small pulmonary emboli.

Pulmonary embolus is one of the most commonly missed diagnoses in the A&E department. The classical triad of pleuritic chest pain, dyspnoea and haemoptysis is not often seen. Clinical signs such as a raised jugular venous pressure and a loud second heart sound may not be present and the S1 Q3 T3 pattern on the ECG is rare. One must remain alert to the possibility of the diagnosis and perform blood gases on any case in which you consider the diagnosis a possibility.

Case 14

1 Stenosing tenovaginitis of thumb (trigger thumb).
2 Refer to plastic or hand surgeon for operative treatment.

Trigger thumb is a relatively common condition which usually presents in young infants between the ages of 6 months and 2 years. It is a developmental abnormality in which the sheath of the flexor pollicis longus tendon is thickened and there is a constricting fibrocartilaginous band at the level of the metacarpophalangeal joint. When the child flexes the finger the thickened tendon becomes bunched behind the constricting band, resulting in loss of extension at the interphalangeal joint. The bunched tendon can often be palpated as a tender nodule over the palmar surface of the metacarpophalangeal joint.

Treatment of this condition is surgical. The patient should be referred to a hand surgeon for operation under a general anaesthetic. Excision of a small piece of the constricting band is curative.

A similar condition, trigger finger, is frequently seen in the finger tendons in adult life. This may respond to local steroid injection, avoiding the need for surgery.

Case 15

1 Immobilization of the patient's neck.
2 Proceed with ventricular fibrillation protocol.
Rewarm the patient using active internal methods.

This patient had arrived at the department in cardiac arrest secondary to near drowning. The possible causes of this episode should not be overlooked. Cervical spine injury can easily result from a dive into a shallow pool. This patient should therefore have had his cervical spine immobilized using a rigid collar, sandbags and tape whilst his airway was being assessed. Immersion in cold water leads to rapid development of hypothermia. A rectal temperature should be recorded on all patients who have had a significant immersion in water. Other conditions that may have resulted in the near-drowning episode such as drug overdose and myocardial infarction should also be excluded.

This patient should be managed according to the ventricular fibrillation protocol of the European Resuscitation Council, commencing with defibrillation at 200 J. However, defibrillation is unlikely to be successful until the patient's temperature is above

30°C. Core rewarming should be instituted as soon as possible. The ideal method is by using extracorporeal circulation such as cardiac bypass together with a blood warmer. However this is unlikely to be available in most departments. Other methods that can be used are warmed humidified air, warmed intravenous fluids (to 40°C) and lavage, whether pleural, gastric, peritoneal or bladder, with warm fluids. There is no proved benefit from the use of steroids or barbiturates. Resuscitation may be prolonged whilst the patient's temperature is raised above 30°C. The patient should not be pronounced dead until defibrillation is unsuccessful at this temperature.

This patient was warmed using warm intravenous fluids and pleural lavage. He was defibrillated back into sinus rhythm when his core temperature was 31°C. Subsequent investigation showed that he had suffered a widepread anterior myocardial infarction. Unfortunately he subsequently developed adult respiratory distress syndrome (ARDS) and died 5 days later.

Case 16

1 Admit the patient for 24 hours and give H_2-antagonist, then repeat X-ray.
2 Yes, patient could be discharged with lactulose and advised to return if cell has not been excreted after 7 days.
3 Those that contain mercury, are large and are new.

Miniature button batteries are being increasingly used in electrical appliances in and around the home. Their size and availability result in a large number of children being seen each year following accidental ingestion. Other groups that may swallow batteries include the psychiatrically ill and the elderly who may confuse a battery (often from their hearing aid) with their medication.

Management depends on three factors – first, the site at which the battery has lodged, second the type of battery and finally the number of batteries. A chest and abdominal X-ray should be performed to determine that a battery has indeed been ingested and to locate its position in the gastrointestinal tract. All batteries that have lodged in the oesophagus should be removed because of the high risk of oesophageal perforation. If the battery has passed through to the stomach then the risk of complication reduces. These patients should be admitted and given H_2-antagonists to decrease stomach acidity and therefore corrosion of the battery. With adults metoclopramide should also be given to promote gastric emptying. The patient should then be X-rayed again after 24 hours. If the battery has passed the pylorus the patient can be discharged on laxatives. If, however, it remains in the stomach and is of a mercury type it should be removed. This can either be achieved using a gastroscope or sometimes with a powerful magnet. It is rarely necessary to proceed to laparotomy. Non-mercury batteries can be left in the stomach for another 24 hours before removal becomes a necessity.

If the battery has already passed through the pylorus at initial presentation, the patient can be discharged on laxatives. The parents should be instructed to sieve the child's faeces and return after a week if the cell has not passed.

Batteries are dangerous for several reasons. Most contain corrosive alkali in high concentrations. Mucosal burns are also caused by electrical currents that are set up around the cell. New batteries are therefore more dangerous than those that are nearly electrically discharged. Mercury batteries are especially dangerous because of the presence of mercuric oxide. This is a corrosive in itself but can also lead to mercury toxicity. Large batteries cause more problems as they have a higher tendency to lodge in the upper gastrointestinal tract. Finally, multiple batteries will result in increased risk and should be removed if lodged in the stomach.

Reference

Thompson N, Lowe-Ponsford F, Mant TGK, Volans GN (1990) Button battery ingestion: a review. *Adverse Drug React. Acute Poisoning Rev.* **9**: 157–182

Case 17

1 Cardiac causes:
    Atrial fibrillation.
    Silent myocardial infarction.
    Postural hypotension.
  Neurological causes:
    Vertebrobasilar insufficiency.
    Stroke.
    Transient ischaemic attack.
  Infective causes:
    Urinary tract infection.
    Chest infection.
  Iatrogenic causes:
    Electrolyte imbalance.
    'Hangover' effect from hypnotic.

2 12-lead ECG.

Chest X-ray.

X-ray pelvis and both hips.

FBC, urea and electrolytes and blood sugar.

Cardiac enzymes.

Ward test of urine and midstream specimen of urine (MSU).

3 Collapse in the elderly is a difficult clinical problem. There are a multitude of causes and multisystem pathology may be present. However, if the problem is approached in a systematic manner the task becomes easier. Cardiovascular and neurological events and infection are the most common causes of collapse. Myocardial infarction should be excluded with serial ECGs and cardiac enzymes. Cardiac arrhythmias may not be evident on initial presentation and may require longer-term monitoring. A cardiac cause that should not be missed is postural hypotension. Standing and lying blood pressure should be checked in all these patients. Neurological causes include cerebrovascular accidents as well as more transitory causes of loss of consciousness such as transient ischaemic attacks or epileptic fits. A careful neurological assessment should be made. Neck movement (which may provoke vertebrobasilar insufficiency) should be assessed and the carotids auscultated for bruits.

Infection of the urinary tract should be excluded with an MSU and a chest X-ray obtained to look for evidence of infection, cardiac failure and occult pathology.

Medication may precipitate collapse, for instance chronic use of naproxen leading to gastric erosions and anaemia. Finally there may be underlying disease such as a hidden malignancy or unrecognized hypothyroidism.

The true diagnosis of most of these patients cannot be determined in the A&E department. The A&E doctor should make an assessment of the patient and arrange the investigations that he or she feels may lead to the correct diagnosis. It is quite acceptable to refer the patient to the inpatient team without a definitive diagnosis. This may not become apparent until much later.

The final diagnosis in this case was atrial fibrillation precipitated by a urinary tract infection. She was also noted to have a fractured left superior pubic ramus. She was discharged home 1 week later when her atrial fibrillation and cardiac failure had settled after treatment of her urinary tract infection. The nitrazepam was stopped as this was felt to have contributed to her collapse. Social service support with a daily home help and meals on wheels was arranged for a period of 6 weeks whilst she recovered from the bony injury.

Case 18

1 Threatened miscarriage.
2 Reassure patient.
  Arrange ultrasound to confirm diagnosis.
  Advise rest at home.

Abortion or miscarriage is loss of a fetus before 24 weeks of gestation. Over 20% of pregnancies miscarry, most in the first trimester, so the condition is seen quite commonly in A&E departments. Initial assessment should concentrate on the ABCs. In some cases haemorrhage will be large and fluid and blood replacement necessary.

The major clinical difficulty is to exclude the diagnosis of ectopic pregnancy. The symptoms can be very similar, with abdominal pain and bleeding, and differentiation cannot always be made on symptoms and signs alone. The investigation of choice is ultrasound. This can be performed either transabdominally or transvaginally. The presence of a fetus with an active heart in the uterus confirms the diagnosis of a threatened miscarriage. If the uterus is empty, an ectopic pregnancy should be strongly suspected and the patient referred for laparoscopy.

Seventy-five per cent of patients with a threatened abortion will settle. Their blood group should be checked and they should be given anti-D if Rhesus-negative. They should be advised to rest at home and abstain from coitus.

If the cervical os is open, the diagnosis is inevitable abortion. The patient should be admitted for a dilatation and curettage to remove any remaining fetal or chorionic tissue. A missed abortion occurs when the fetus dies but is retained. The diagnosis can be made with ultrasound, when the fetus will be seen to be dead and the uterus small-for-dates.

Case 19

1 Postconcussion headache.
2 Reassurance and explanation of cause.
  Simple analgesia.
3 Symptoms:
      Persistent vomiting.
      Sudden onset of pain.
  Signs:
      Abnormal pupillary reactions.
      Decrease in Glasgow Coma Score.
      Any focal neurological deficit.

Numerous patients with many different headache syndromes present to the A&E department. Most of these patients will have benign conditions but it is important to recognize the clinical features that may indicate significant pathology.

This patient has a classical history of a postconcussion headache. The headache usually involves the whole head and is associated with symptoms of light-headedness, malaise, irritability, anxiety and fatigue. These symptoms may persist for weeks and occasionally longer. The patient should be reassured that these symptoms are common after a head injury and will resolve with time. Simple analgesics should be given.

There are certain symptoms that should always be treated with caution in a patient with a headache. Acute onset should always raise the possibility of a subarachnoid haemorrhage. If vomiting persists in a patient after a head injury it may be a sign of intracranial haematoma. Double vision and visual disturbances are common after head injuries and cannot usually be substantiated with testing. However, if there is any real neurological deficit demonstrable, a CT scan should be performed. Finally, change in behaviour or personality may be mentioned by a relative. This subtle sign may be the only indication of a small intracerebral bleed.

Case 20

1 Chin lift.
  Jaw thrust.
  Oropharyngeal airway.
  Nasopharyngeal airway.
  Laryngeal mask.
2 Right-sided tension pneumothorax.
  Needle thoracocentesis with large bore cannula in second interspace midclavicular line.
3 Reassess patient for response to intervention.
  Assess circulation.

The Advanced Trauma Life Support system (ATLS) emphasizes a safe system for managing the trauma patient. The tenets of this system are to assess and also treat life-threatening conditions as they are found in a logical order. One should always commence with the airway and cervical spine. If the airway is obstructed simple manoeuvres should be tried first. Chin lift or jaw thrust may succeed but can be difficult to hold for a long time. In these cases an oropharyngeal airway may be suitable. If the patient cannot tolerate a

Guedel airway, he or she may accept a nasopharyngeal airway, which impinges less on the back of the pharynx.

Other adjuncts that should be available for simple airway management are suction and Magill's forceps to remove vomitus and foreign bodies. A device that has recently been introduced into emergency care is the laryngeal mask. Its main advantage is that it is easy to use and can provide an adequate airway in most unconscious patients. However, it does not protect the airway from aspiration. It may be useful when difficulty is being encountered in maintaining a patient's airway and expertise is not immediately available to perform endotracheal intubation.

The diagnosis of a tension pneumothorax should always be clinical and prompt the rapid insertion of a wide-bore cannula into the second intercostal space in the midclavicular line of the affected side. Whenever an intervention is performed one should reassess the patient to ensure that there has been improvement. The next stage would be to assess circulation using pulse rate, blood pressure and capillary return, take blood and commence intravenous fluids through two wide-bore cannulae. One should also ask an assistant to set up a tray for a chest drain, which should be inserted as soon as possible as definitive treatment of the pneumothorax. If ever the patient starts to deteriorate, one should return to the beginning and start again.

DATA INTERPRETATION QUESTIONS

Table 1 Normal values

Blood gases	
P_{O_2}	11–14.5 kPa
pH	7.36–7.44
P_{CO_2}	4.8–6.0 kPa
Base excess	−2 to +2
Urea and electrolytes	
Na^+	135–145 mmol/l
K^+	3.6–5.2 mmol/l
Urea	3.0–7.0 mmol/l
HCO_3^-	22–30 mmol/l
Cl^-	95–105 mmol/l

Data Interpretation

The A&E physician will see many patients during a single shift of duty. There are certain investigations that can be performed that aid either in diagnosis or in treatment of the patient. The result of the investigation should be available within an hour if it is to be useful in patient management. This limits the spectrum of tests that can be performed.

At present simple haematological and biochemical investigations such as FBC, ESR, U&Es, amylase and blood glucose may be performed. Emergency blood gas analysis should be available in most departments. Microscopy of urine, blood and swabs may also be undertaken. With the advent of more automated systems and near-patient testing, it will be possible in the future to have a much wider spectrum of investigation available to the emergency physician.

The emergency physician should usually only order investigations when he or she can act upon the result. If he or she orders other investigations, for example as courtesy to an admitting team, he or she should ensure that an identified person will locate the result and then take any necessary action.

Data interpretation questions

Cardiac rhythm strips and 12-lead ECGs can be performed quickly. Together with blood gas results these investigations cause the majority of difficulties with data interpretation in the A&E department. This section concentrates on methods of approaching these problems.

Cardiac rhythms

Rhythm strip interpretation is a skill that the A&E physician needs to acquire. Remember that the strip should be used to comment on cardiac rhythm alone. The reading from a single lead will not give enough information to comment on the ST segments or T waves. The best lead to use is standard lead II (negative lead over right clavicle, positive lead over left lower chest). This gives a good representation of the P wave and of the QRS complex. Lead V1 also shows atrial activity well.

Most rhythms can be quickly recognized using a simple system. This is the method that we use:

Step 1: Check the pulse
Rhythm interpretation should always commence with a pulse check. The clinical state of the patient is of paramount importance. Without this step, the diagnosis of cardiac arrest (particularly if the patient is in electromechanical dissociation) may be missed.

Step 2: Is this a rhythm that I easily recognize?
Sinus rhythm can be identified after rapid inspection. Dangerous rhythms such as ventricular fibrillation and asystole should also be identified by pattern recognition and the necessary prompt treatment instituted. If the rhythm is not recognized then proceed to step 3.

Step 3: What is the ventricular rate?
The ventricular rate can be calculated by counting the number of large squares between two consecutive complexes and then dividing this number into 300. (The paper runs at 25 mm/s and one big square is 5 mm.) This can be simply represented as in Table 2.

If the rhythm is irregular, count the distance between five complexes and divide into 1500. Do not always rely on a cardiac monitor to give the correct rate. Incorrect setting of the gain may result in the rate being erroneously high or low.

Table 2 A quick way to calculate ventricular rates

Squares between QRSs	Ventricular rate
1	300
2	150
3	100
4	75
5	60
6	50
7	43

Step 4: Is the basic ventricular rhythm regular or irregular?
This may be ascertained on quick inspection or may require careful
mapping out with a pen and paper. If the rhythm is irregular one
should decide if it is regularly irregular or irregularly irregular. Atrial
fibrillation is the most common cause of an irregularly irregular
pulse. Other causes such as atrial flutter with variable heart block
should also be considered.

Causes of a regularly irregular rhythm include the sinus arrhythmia
of normal respiration and Wenckebach (Möbitz type I) second degree
heart block.

A rhythm that is basically regular may have areas of irregularity
caused by extra beats. If these occur prior to the next expected beat
they are known as a *premature* beat. If they occur late (i.e. because a
beat of the normal rhythm has been missed), then they are called
escape beats.

*Step 5: Are there P waves and do they bear a constant relationship
to the QRS complexes?*
Look for P waves, indicating atrial contraction. If you cannot identify
any, then look for the sawtooth flutter waves of atrial flutter. If
neither is present and the rhythm is irregularly irregular then the
diagnosis is almost certainly atrial fibrillation.

If P waves are present look at their relationship with the QRS
complexes. If the relationship is constant check that the distance
between the P wave and the QRS complex is less than 0.2/s (one
large square). If the distance is greater then the patient is in
first-degree heart block.

If the relationship is constant but some P waves are not followed
by QRS complexes, then the diagnosis is Möbitz type II
second-degree heart block.

147

RHYTHM STRIP: II
25 mm/sec; 1 cm/mV

.05-40Hz   24586

Question 1

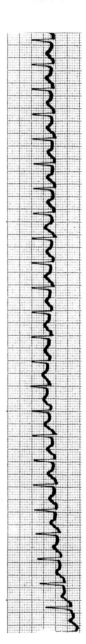

Question 2

If the relationship is variable with the distance between each successive P wave and its following QRS complex increasing until there is a P wave without a QRS complex, then the diagnosis is Wenckebach second-degree heart block.

If there is no constant relationship between the P waves and the QRS complexes then the rhythm is third-degree heart block.

Step 6: Is the QRS complex narrow or broad
The normal QRS complex should be less than 0.12/s long (three small squares). If this is the case and the rhythm is fast, it should be described as a narrow-complex tachycardia. This will have originated from or above the atrioventricular node. If the complexes are broad, the rhythm may have originated either from the ventricle or from the atria if aberrant electrical conduction is present.

If the rhythm is still not apparent one should look for more information. This can be provided by the 12-lead ECG or by looking at a longer rhythm strip. Some difficult rhythms may need intracardiac electrophysiology for their correct determination.

Rhythm strip interpretation questions

Question 1
This is the rhythm strip taken from a 25-year-old woman. She noticed a sudden onset of fast regular palpitations whilst out shopping. The palpitations have been present for 50 minutes. She has had one previous similar episode in the past. This resolved spontaneously and was not investigated. She does not take any medication and is otherwise well. Her blood pressure is 110/80 mmHg.

a What is the ventricular rate?
b What is the rhythm?
c How would you treat this patient in the A&E department?

Question 2
This is the rhythm strip taken from a 55-year-old woman. She noticed that she had a fast heart beat when she awoke in the morning. She has not had any previous similar episodes and has no other symptoms apart from the tachycardia. Ten years ago she was diagnosed as having essential hypertension and commenced on bendrofluazide 5 mg/day by her general practitioner. She has been otherwise well. On examination her blood pressure is 130/90 mmHg.

a What is the ventricular rate?
b What is the rhythm?
c What diagnostic test could you perform in the A&E department to confirm this rhythm?

Question 3

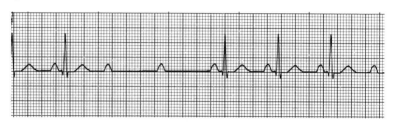

This is the rhythm strip of a 62-year-old man who presented to the A&E department with a 20 minute history of an aching pain in his chest, which developed when watching a football match. The pain receded on arrival in the department. His father died aged 55 from a heart attack. He is a heavy smoker. There is no other relevant history. On examination he has a blood pressure of 140/100 mmHg.

a What other investigation would you like urgently performed?
b What is the ventricular rate?
c What is the rhythm?

Question 4

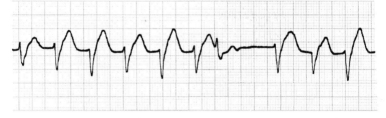

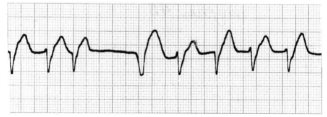

This is the rhythm strip taken from a 60-year-old man who presented to the A&E department with a 2-hour history of central chest pain associated with a feeling of light-headedness. He has suffered with angina for 5 years and uses a GTN spray on average four times a week. On examination he is peripherally cool and his blood pressure is 80/50 mmHg.

a What is the rhythm?
b How would you treat this patient in the A&E department?
c How might your treatment differ if the blood pressure was normal?

Question 5

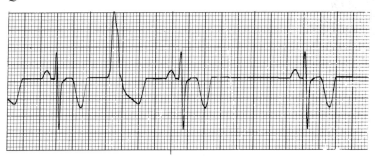

This is the rhythm strip obtained from a cardiac monitor of an 85-year-old woman who was brought into the department after a high-speed car accident. The patient has no pulse. Cardiopulmonary resuscitation is underway.

a What is the diagnosis?
b Name four likely causes of the rhythm in this patient.
c Outline the management of this patient in the A&E department.

Twelve-lead ECG interpretation

The system for interpreting 12-lead ECGs follows on from the rhythm strip interpretation. This is the system that we suggest:

Step 7: Check the ECG has been correctly performed
This can be quickly checked by looking at lead aVR. The P waves, the dominant QRS deflection and the T wave should be upside down. If they are not, this suggests that the ECG has been performed incorrectly. Go and check. Lead aVR can now be ignored.

Step 8: Check the axis
Exact determination of the axis is not necessary in the A&E department. All one needs to know is if the axis is normal, deviated

to the right or deviated to the left. Use this system and look at the dominant deflection of the QRS complex in standard leads I–III.

Upwards in I and II = normal axis
Downwards in I = right axis deviation
Downwards in II = left axis deviation

Step 9: Are the QRS complexes all normal?
Check that all the QRS complexes are less than three small squares wide. If the patient is in sinus rhythm and the complexes are widened and M-shaped in leads V5 and V6, then left bundle branch block is present. If the patient is in left bundle branch block then no further interpretation can be made from the QRS and T waves and the ST segment. If the M-shaped complexes are in V1 and V2 then the patient is likely to have right bundle branch block. Check for the presence of pathological Q waves in the inferior leads, II, III and aVF and in the anterior leads, 1, aVL and V1–V6. Look for the tall R waves of right and left ventricular hypertrophy. Finally, look for the notched QRS complexes seen with the δ waves of the pre-excitation syndromes and the J waves of hypothermia.

Step 10: Inspect the ST segments and the T waves
Start by looking for convex ST elevation in the anterior and inferior leads that may indicate an acute infarct. Look for ST depression that may be a reciprocal change opposite an infarct or may indicate ischaemia. Check that there is no concave ST elevation indicating the diagnosis of pericarditis. Then look at the T waves. Inverted T waves may indicate ischaemia or a recent infarct. Peaked T waves occur in hyperkalaemia.

Step 11: Look for unusual patterns
Finally, check that there are no unusual patterns that you have missed. Look for the S1, Q3, T3 pattern of a large pulmonary embolus and the 'mirror image' changes seen in leads V1 to V3 of the true posterior infarct.

Twelve-Lead ECG interpretation questions

Question 6
This is the ECG of a 75-year-old previously fit woman who came to the A&E department complaining of severe central chest pain which had been present for 1 hour. She described the pain as a tearing radiating through to her back. On examination she was cool and clammy. Her blood pressure was 140/100 mmHg. There were no other abnormalities detected.

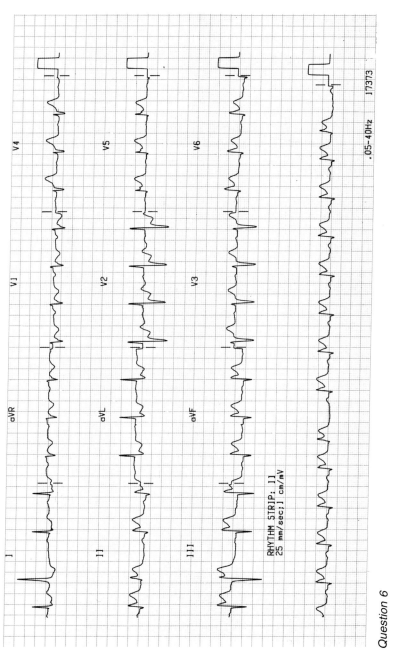

RHYTHM STRIP: II
25 mm/sec; 1 cm/mV

.05-40Hz   17373

Question 6

153

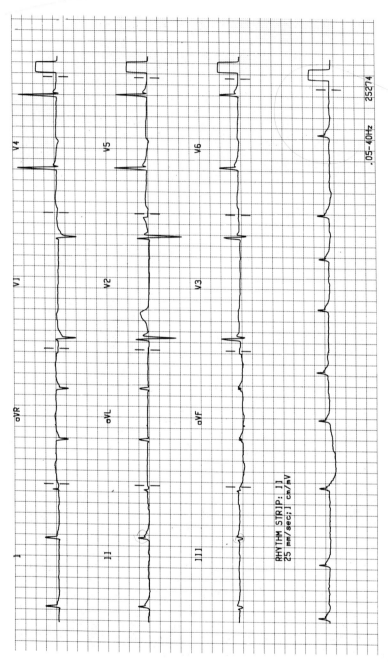

RHYTHM STRIP: II
25 mm/sec; 1 cm/mV

.05-40Hz   25274

Question 7

154

a What is the ECG diagnosis?
b What underlying diagnosis do you suspect?
c How would you confirm this diagnosis?

Question 7
This is the ECG of an 85-year-old woman who had been brought into the A&E department collapsed and unconscious.

a What is the rhythm?
b Name one other abnormal feature present on this ECG.
c What is the diagnosis?

Question 8
A 65-year-old man attends the A&E department with a four-hour history of central crushing chest pain. He has also noticed shortness of breath on exertion for the past four days. His 12-lead ICG is shown.

a Write a report on this ECG.
b What is your differential diagnosis?

Question 9
A 38-year-old man attends the A&E department with a 3-day history of an aching central chest pain. He is a non-smoker and has no family history of ischaemic heart disease. Clinical examination is normal. This is his 12-lead ECG.

a Write a report on this ECG.
b What diagnosis does the ECG suggest?

Question 10
A 37-year-old woman comes to the A&E department complaining of a tight central chest pain. This developed 45 minutes ago whilst she was at an aerobics class. She still has a mild ache in her central chest. Systemic examination is normal.

a What abnormalities are present on this ECG?
b How would you initially manage this patient?

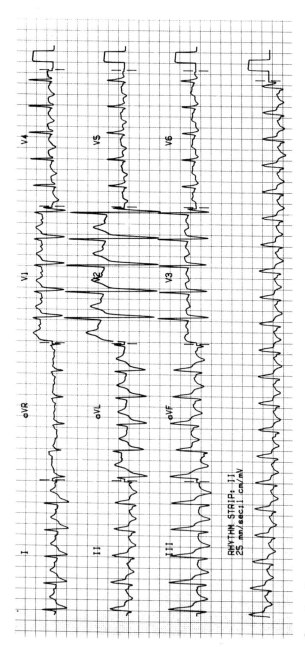

RHYTHM STRIP: II
25 mm/sec; 1 cm/mV

Question 8

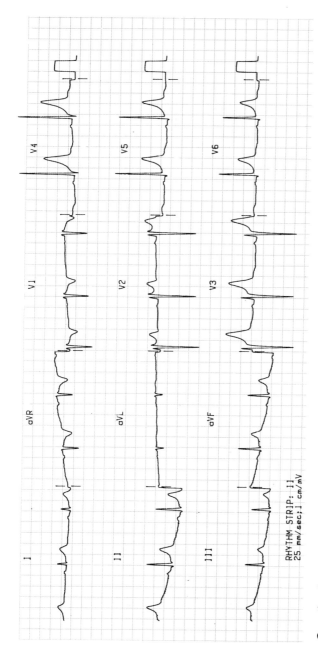

RHYTHM STRIP: II
25 mm/sec; 1 cm/mV

Question 9

157

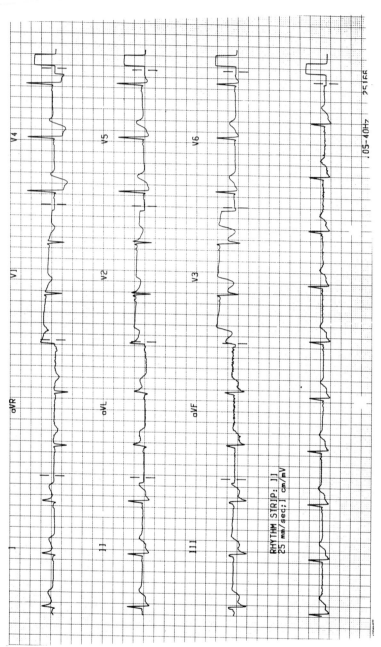

RHYTHM STRIP: II
25 mm/sec; 1 cm/mV

.05-40Hz

Question 10

Blood gas interpretation

Blood gases are one of the most useful investigations available in the A&E department. Blood gas machines are calibrated to give standard results at a normal body temperature. If the patient temperature is not normal then this information should be entered into the machine when the sample is inserted. The results may also be unreliable if abnormal haemoglobins such as carboxyhaemoglobin or methaemoglobin are present as not all gas machines will automatically compensate for these factors.

Blood gas interpretation is made simpler if a simple system is followed:

Step 1: Check the inspired oxygen level
This will not be printed on the result paper so it should be visually checked and then noted down.

Step 2: Check the partial pressure of oxygen
If the value is normal on room air then the patient is not hypoxic. If the value is low on air then the patient is hypoxic. If the value is low on added oxygen then the hypoxia is more severe.

Step 3: Check the pH
If the pH is between 7.36 and 7.44 then it is normal.

Step 4: Check the partial pressure of carbon dioxide
This is a measure of the patient's ventilation. If the level is raised then the patient is underventilating. If the pH was acidotic then this is a respiratory acidosis. If the level is raised but the pH is alkalotic then this is respiratory compensation (i.e. underventilation) for a metabolic acidosis. *alkalosis.*

Step 5: Check the standardized base excess
This is a value calculated by the blood gas machine that represents the metabolic component alone of the acid–base status. If the pH is alkalotic and the base excess is increased the patient has a metabolic alkalosis. If the value is raised but the pH is acidotic then the patient has metabolic compensation for a respiratory acidosis.

Step 6: Go back to the patient
The result of a blood gas determination may often need action. If change is suggested, such as increasing patient ventilation, then a repeat blood gas should be performed after the action has been performed.

159

Data interpretation questions

Question 11
These are the blood gases taken from a 21-year-old woman who noticed that she was short of breath whilst shopping in a supermarket. She is complaining of numbness around her mouth.

Blood gas report: patient breathing room air
P_{O_2} 16.2 kPa
pH   7.50
P_{CO_2} 2.1 kPa
Base excess   −2

a How would you describe this abnormality?
b What is the likely cause?

Question 12
A 21-year-old student was brought to the department by her flatmate who found her in a drowsy and confused state. On examination she is unconscious and hyperventilating. A BM stick reads 6. These are her blood gases:

Blood gas report: patient breathing room air
P_{O_2} 16.9 kPa
pH   7.02
P_{CO_2} 1.6 kPa
Base excess   −16

a How would you describe these abnormalities?
b What is the most likely diagnosis?
c How would you treat this patient?

Question 13
A 24-year-old asthmatic man is brought to the department complaining of severe shortness of breath. He is having difficulty speaking. You immediately commence him on a salbutamol nebulizer run on high-flow oxygen and take a blood gas sample. This is the result:

Blood gas report: patient on high-flow oxygen
P_{O_2} 12.1 kPa
pH   7.30
P_{CO_2} 6.4 kPa
Base excess   −7

a Describe the abnormalities.
b Are these findings consistent with a severe asthma attack?
c How would you treat this patient if he did not improve?

160

Question 14
A 15-year-old young woman is brought into the department in a very weak and debilitated state. These are her blood gases.

Blood gas result: patient on room air
P_{O_2} 11.0 kPa
pH   7.47
P_{CO_2} 7.2 kPa
Base excess   + 10

a What is the primary acid–base disorder in this case?
b Suggest an underlying cause.

Question 15
A 75-year-old man is brought in to the A&E department by ambulance. He had called the ambulance when he had become acutely short of breath. The ambulance technician started him on 60% oxygen and brought him to the hospital. He is now unable to speak and no other history is available. On examination he has nicotine stained fingers. His pulse is bounding at a rate of 120 beats/min. He has a respiratory rate of 32 breaths/min and on examining his barrel shaped chest you can hear the occasional wheeze. A chest X-ray shows overinflated lungs but no pneumothorax. These are his blood gas results:

Blood gas report: patient on 60% oxygen
P_{O_2} 7.1 kPa
pH   7.17
P_{CO_2} 9.4 kPa
Base excess   −10

a Describe the abnormalities.
b What diagnosis would you suspect?
c What would be your immediate action?

Miscellaneous data interpretations

Question 16
A 74-year-old man presents to the A&E department with a painful swollen knee. He remembers knocking the knee against a low table the previous day. On examination he is apyrexial. There is a moderate knee effusion and flexion of the knee is painful. X-ray of the knee does not reveal any fracture. The knee was aspirated and this is the report phoned from the laboratory:

Data interpretation questions

Knee aspirate
Turbid fluid, neutrophils ++
Weakly positive birefringent crystals ++

a What is the likely diagnosis?
b What abnormality may have been noted on close inspection of the knee X-ray?

Question 17

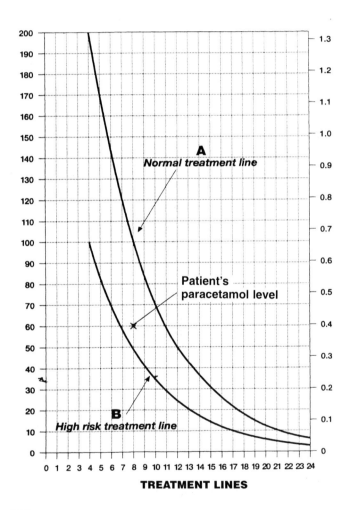

A 46-year-old alcoholic man comes to the department after taking an overdose of paracetamol. He says he took 40 paracetamol about 8 hours ago. His blood paracetamol level is shown on the paracetamol treatment nomogram.

a Would you give this patient a gastric lavage?
b Would you give this patient activated charcoal?
c How would you treat this patient's overdose?

Question 18
A 74-year-old man presents to the department complaining of severe thirst. He is diabetic but is controlled on diet alone. On examination he is mildly confused and has a temperature of 38°C. His skin is dry and he appears severely dehydrated. These are the results of his urea and electrolytes, blood sugar and urine testing.

Urea and electrolytes
Na^+ 158 mmol/l
K^+ 5.0 mmol/l
Urea   17 mmol/l

Blood sugar: 52 mmol/l

Urine: glucose +++ , ketones negative.

a What is the likely diagnosis?
b How would you treat this patient?

Question 19
A 55-year-old man is brought into the department having a grand mal seizure. This is controlled with intravenous diazepam. His urine is noted to look very concentrated. Blood is sent for estimation of urea and electrolytes and glucose. These are the results.
Urea and electrolytes
Na^+ 114 mmol/l
K^+ 4.0 mmol/l
Urea   3.9 mmol/l

Blood glucose: 4.1 mmol/l

a What is the likely pathological process causing these abnormalities?
b Name two causes of this pathological process.

Data interpretation questions

Question 20
A 45-year-old homeless man was brought into the hospital in a
drowsy and confused state. He was a known alcoholic. On
examination he was apyrexial. He had numerous spider naevi. He
was drowsy and disoriented in time and place but further examination
of the central and peripheral nervous system was normal. A full
blood count, urea and electrolytes, blood sugar, blood alcohol and
blood gases are reported as follows:

FBC: Hb 12.2 g/dl, WCC 11.4 $\times 10^9$/l, Platelets 181 $\times 10^9$/l
U & Es: Na$^+$ 135 mmol/l, K$^+$ 4 mmol/l, Cl$^-$ 95 mmol/l, HCO$_3^-$
     10 mmol/l, urea 8.2 mmol/l
Blood glucose: 3.5 mmol/l
Blood alcohol: 40m g/dl
Urine ketones: negative

a What is the most likely diagnosis?
b How would you treat this condition?

DATA INTERPRETATION ANSWERS

Question 1

a The ventricular rate is about 215 beats/min.

b A regular narrow-complex (supraventricular) tachycardia.

c Give oxygen and establish IV access.
Try a vagal manoeuvre. If no response:
Adenosine bolus 3 mg then 6 mg then 12 mg then 12 mg. If no response:
Call for expert help.

There are two main types of narrow-complex tachycardia – those caused by rapid atrial activity such as atrial tachycardia and those where an additional connection is present between the atria and ventricles, the atrioventricular re-entrant tachycardias. Atrial tachycardia occurs with digoxin toxicity, ischaemic heart disease and cardiomyopathy. In a young fit person who is tolerating the rhythm well, atrioventricular re-entrant tachycardia is the most likely diagnosis. The re-entrant tachycardias can be further subdivided into those where the extra pathway is in the node – the **atrioventricular nodal re-entrant tachycardias** – and those where there is an accessory pathway the **atrioventricular re-entrant tachycardias**.

The Resuscitation Council (UK) has recently published guidelines for the management of narrow-complex tachycardia (Algorithm 1).

After establishing IV access and giving oxygen, a vagal manoeuvre should be tried. The Valsalva manoeuvre is probably the best method. This involves forcefully expiring for 10–15 seconds against a closed nose and mouth. Alternatively, firm pressure can be applied over one carotid artery for 5 seconds. This should be avoided in patients with carotid bruits. If these methods fail, then adenosine should be given. It has a very short half-life so should be injected rapidly. The patient should be warned of a transient feeling of facial flushing and dyspnoea. If 3 mg of adenosine fails then further doses of 6, 12 and 12 mg should be given at 1–2 minute intervals. With this dosage regimen, over 90% of the re-entrant tachcardias will be converted back to sinus rhythm. The drug should be avoided in patients with a history of asthma and those taking dipyridamole.

Adenosine acts by blocking conduction at the atrioventricular node. Consequently it can cause ventricular standstill which may last for 10

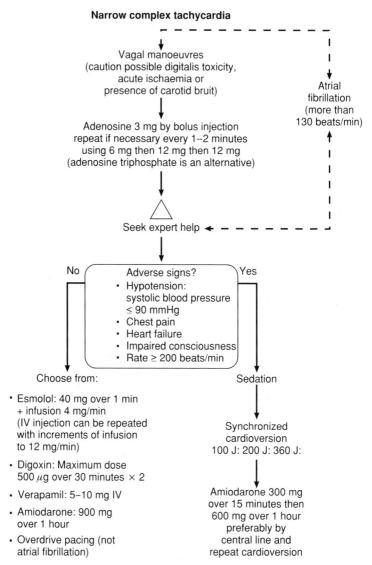

Algorithm 1 Treatment of sustained supraventricular tachycardia. Reproduced with permission from the European Resuscitation Council.

seconds or longer. If it does not work, senior advice should be sought. Other methods of treatment may need to be instituted such as cardioversion, the use of drugs such as verapamil or amiodarone or overdrive pacing.

When the patient has reverted back to sinus rhythm, a full 12-lead ECG should be inspected for evidence of an accessory pathway. The patient should be referred to the cardiological team for further investigation of the cause of the rhythm.

The tachycardia in this patient was terminated with a bolus of 12 mg adenosine. She was referred to the cardiologists who, using intracardiac electrophysiological techniques, discovered an accessory pathway. This was ablated using radiofrequency energy. She has had no further recurrences of the tachycardia.

Question 2
a The ventricular rate is 150 beats/min.
b Narrow complex tachycardia, probably atrial flutter with two to one block.
c Give adenosine 3 mg and observe the rhythm.

A narrow complex tachycardia with a ventricular rate that stays around 150 beats/min is highly sugggestive of the diagnosis of atrial flutter with two to one atrioventricular block. Atrial flutter is usually associated with coronary or hypertensive heart disease. Other causes include alcohol abuse, rheumatic heart disease and the cardiomyopathies. It can be paroxysmal or sustained and is usually initiated by an atrial extrasystole. The flutter is caused by a re-entrant circuit, usually within the right atrium. The atrial rate is usually about 300 beats/min. The ventricular response is determined by the conducting ability of the atrioventricular node. Commonly each second flutter wave is conducted, leading to a ventricular rate of 150 beats/min. The flutter or F wave has a characteristic sawtooth baseline and is best seen in standard leads II, III or AVF. If lead V1 is inspected, the F wave may appear in more discrete form.

Adenosine can be used to slow conduction transiently through the atrioventricular node. A printout of the rhythm strip should be activated as the rhythm transformation will only be transitory and can be easily missed. Dosage should again start at 3 mg. A sawtooth pattern of atrial flutter was revealed in this patient when 6 mg of Adenosine was given.

The aim of treatment of atrial flutter of acute onset should be to restore the patient back to normal sinus rhythm. The patient should be referred to the inpatient medical team. Direct current cardioversion is very effective in restoring sinus rhythm in these patients. If cardioversion fails, other treatments such as rapid atrial pacing or drugs such as flecainide may be tried. If normal rhythm cannot be restored then the ventricular rate should be controlled with drugs such as digoxin.

This woman was cardioverted back into sinus rhythm using 50 V direct current. She was commenced on sotalol to prevent recurrence of the arrhythmia.

Question 3
a A 12-lead ECG.
b The ventricular rate is 50 beats/min.
c The rhythm is Möbitz type II second-degree heart block.

This patient is bradycardic secondary to Möbitz type II second-degree heart block with irregular conduction of p waves. Myocardial infarction was subsequently revealed by the 12-lead ECG. A temporary pacing wire was inserted by the on-call medical team prior to the patient receiving streptokinase. His block progressed to complete heart block despite the thrombolytic therapy so a permanent pacemaker was inserted 5 days later.

In second-degree heart block there is intermittent failure of condution of atrial activity through to the ventricles. With Möbitz type II block there is no antecedent progressive lengthening of the PR interval before the dropped ventricular beats. Ventricular activity in Möbitz type II block can be regular, such as with two to one conduction of atrial beats, or irregular with no pattern of dropped beats. The atrial rate usually remains regular.

Möbitz type II block usually occurs due to impaired conduction in the bundle of His or bundle branches and so the QRS complexes are often wide. As the block is lower, the outlook is more sinister than with Wenckebach second-degree heart block. There is a significant incidence of progression to complete heart block and sudden death.

NB: It is quite easy to misinterpret complete heart block as second degree heart block (either Wenckebach or Möbitz type II) if only a cursory glance is taken at the rhythm strip. It is always wise to map out the relationship of the P waves with the QRS complexes to ensure that this mistake is not made.

Question 4
a Broad-complex tachycardia – ventricular tachycardia.
b Give oxygen and establish IV access.
  Seek expert help.

Sedate and cardiovert at 100 J increasing to 200 then 300 J if there is no response.

c Use lignocaine 50 mg over 2 minutes repeated every 5 minutes up to a total dose of 200 mg and start a lignocaine infusion of 2 mg/min.

Give potassium and magnesium if the potassium is known to be low.

The rhythm is a broad-complex tachycardia. Capture and fusion beats can be seen, confirming that the diagnosis is in fact a ventricular tachycardia. A capture beat looks like a normal QRS and occurs when an atrial impulse is conducted normally, activating the ventricle before the abnormal discharge from the ventricular focus. A fusion beat looks bizarre and occurs when a normal complex is superimposed on the beat from the ventricular focus. If P waves can be seen 'walking through' the ventricular complexes, the diagnosis of ventricular tachycardia can again be confirmed (see ECG). Other methods of discerning the two rhythms are less reliable. If there is any doubt in the cause of the rhythm, then treat the patient as if the rhythm is ventricular tachycardia.

A patient who has a wide-complex tachycardia of unknown origin, who is haemodynamically stable and who has not had a recent infarct may be given adenosine as an aid to rhythm recognition. If the rhythm is supraventricular with aberrant conduction it may well convert back to sinus. If it is ventricular nothing will happen.

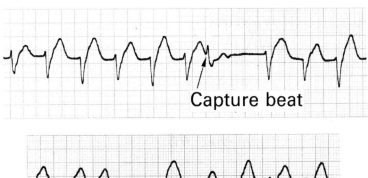
Capture beat

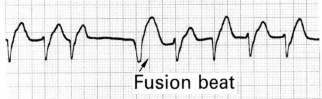
Fusion beat

Data interpretation answers

The treatment algorithm for ventricular tachycardia is as shown in Algorithm 2. The prime factor in the treatment of patients is clinical status. If they are haemodynamically stable, cardioversion with drugs can be attempted. If they are unstable then electrical cardioversion should be used. If there is no pulse the patient should be treated as for ventricular fibrillation.

This man had a low blood pressure. After being given oxygen he was cardioverted with 100 J synchronized direct current shock back into sinus rhythm. A subsequent ECG showed a small anterior subendocardial infarct.

Question 5
a Electromechanical dissociation.
b Hypoxia.
  Tension pneumothorax.
  Hypovolaemia.
  Cardiac tamponade.
c Think of and exclude the possible causes of electromechanical dissociation in this patient.
  Optimize the cardiopulmonary resuscitation by intubating the patient, obtaining IV access and giving adrenaline 1 mg.

The electrical rhythm of this patient is sinus rhythm with a ventricular premature beat. As the patient has no pulse the diagnosis is electromechanical dissociation. Attention should be aimed at providing good cardiopulmonary resusciation. This can be optimized by giving regular adrenaline. The causes of electromechanical dissociation can be divided into those that result from uncoupling of electrical excitation and mechanical contraction and those secondary to mechanical causes. In this patient hypoxia from airway obstruction is an example of the first group and tension pneumothorax, hypovolaemia and cardiac tamponade are examples of mechanical causes.

This patient had a right-sided tension pnemothorax and placement of a large cannula in the second intercostal space was accompanied by the return of a good pulse.

Question 6
a Acute inferolateral myocardial infarction.
b Dissection of the ascending aorta.
c Arrange arch aortogram.

The ECG shows ST elevation in the inferior (II, III and aVF) and lateral (V5 and V6) leads consistent with an acute inferolateral infarct. Deep Q waves have already developed in leads III and aVF, showing that full-thickness damage to the myocardial wall has already occurred.

This patient might be considered a candidate for thrombolysis. However, the history that the patient describes is not consistent with the diagnosis of acute myocardial infarction. A tearing pain radiating through to the back should alert the clinician to the possibility of aortic dissection. The patient should be re-examined for signs of

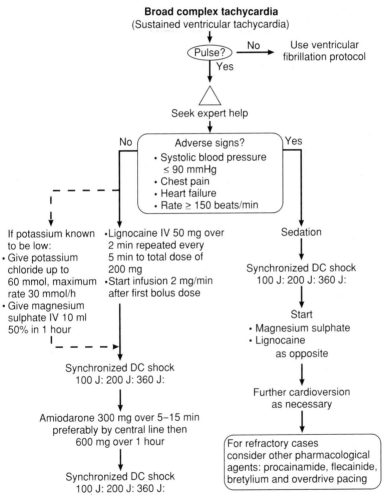

Algorithm 2 Treatment of algorithm for sustained ventricular tachycardia. Reproduced with permission from the European Resuscitation Council.

inequality of pulse or blood pressure between the arms. A chest X-ray will often show widening of the mediastinum. Other abnormalities that may be present include obliteration of the aortic knob, deviation of the trachea to the right and the presence of a pleural cap. The investigation of choice to exclude this diagnosis is an arch aortogram. This will demonstrate the torn intimal flap as a lucent line and the true and false channel. CT scan is an alternative but is less sensitive.

This patient was admitted to the coronary care unit. An arch aortogram confirmed the diagnosis of a dissection of the ascending aorta. Shortly afterwards the patient developed an acute left hemiplegia and died. Post-mortem showed that the dissection had spread proximally to involve the right coronary artery and distally to involve the innominate artery.

Question 7

a Slow atrial fibrillation.
b J waves best seen in leads I, II and V6.
c Hypothermia with atrial fibrillation.

Hypothermia is defined as a core body temperature below 35°C. This should be measured with a low-reading rectal thermometer. At temperatures below 30°C the hypothermia can be defined as severe. The cardiac rhythm changes from a sinus bradycardia to slow atrial fibrillation through ventricular fibrillation to asystole as the temperature decreases. Ventricular fibrillation may be precipitated by movement alone, so the patient should be kept as still as possible.

Management should first address the airway. breathing and circulation. The patient should be removed from the cold environment and possible causes of the hypothermic episode such as alcohol ingestion or sepsis must be sought. The method of rewarming will depend on the severity of the hypothermia and the urgency of resuscitation. Passive external methods such as use of a warm room with warm blankets can be used for mild hypothermia. In the scenario of a cardiac arrest defibrillation may not be successful until the core temperature has been raised to 30°C so more active core rewarming methods are necessary. These include infusing warm peritoneal or pleural lavage fluids and using cardiopulmonary bypass.

The J wave, a small deflection on the downstroke of the QRS complex, is pathognomonic of hypothermia. Prolongation of the QT interval and the PR interval (in those with P waves) also occurs, but these effects are proportional to the degree of bradycardia. Baseline flutter may be seen as the patient warms up and shivering recommences.

This woman had tripped and fallen at home one winter evening and lain overnight on the floor. Her core temperature on arrival was 27°C. She was treated with passive rewarming methods aiming for a 1°C rise per hour. Her rhythm returned to sinus when her temperature was 35°C.

Question 8

a Rate: 115 beats/min.
　　Rhythm: Sinus tachycardia.
　　Q waves present in II, III and aVF
　　ST elevation in II, III and aVF
　　T waves inverted in II, III, aVF, V4, V5 and V6
b Recent inferior myocardial infarction
　　Pulmonary embolism.

This ECG shows changes consistent with a recent inferior myocardial infarction. Deep Q waves are already present in leads III and aVF, indicating full thickness myocardial damage. The T waves are inverted suggesting that the infarct is more than 12 hours old.

This ECG could also be interpreted as showing the SI QIII TIII pattern of a pulmonary embolus. However, the findings in the other two inferior leads (II, aVF) indicate the true diagnosis.

Remember that the diagnosis of pulmonary embolism is easily missed if the condition is not considered. The first change on the ECG is usually a sinus tachycardia. As increasing strain is placed on the right ventricle, right bundle branch block and the pattern of right ventricular hypertrophy and strain are seen (tall R waves with T-wave inversion in the right ventricular leads).

The SI QIII TIII pattern is only seen with a moderate to large pulmonary embolus.

This gentleman was admitted to coronary care but unfortunately sustained a cardiac arrest and died. Post mortem findings showed total occlusion of the right coronary artery with thrombus.

Question 9

a Rate: 92 beats/min.
　　Rhythm: Sinus rhythm.
　　Axis: Normal.
　　QRS complexes: Normal.
　　ST segments and T waves: Concave ST elevation in leads I, II, aVL, aVF and V1–V6.
　　Conclusion: Sinus rhythm with widespread concave ST elevation.
b Acute pericarditis.

Acute pericarditis occurs most commonly in healthy people between the ages of 20 and 40. In these patients it is usually caused by a viral infection. Other causes include bacterial and fungal infections, systemic illnesses such as rheumatic fever and sarcoidosis, trauma, myocardial infarction and drugs. In a significant number of patients the cause remains undiscovered. The patient classically describes a sharp midline pain which is worse on moving and deep inspiration. Leaning forward often eases the pain. On examination a pericardial friction rub, if present, will confirm the diagnosis.

This patient was referred to the on-call medical team who treated him with non-steroidal anti-inflammatory drugs. Paired viral titres showed that the pericarditis was caused by an adenovirus infection.

Question 10

a ST segment elevation in leads I and aVL.
   ST segment depression in leads II, III, aVF and leads V2, V3, V4 and V5.
b Give the patient oxygen.
   Give pain relief with intravenous opiate and antiemetic.
   Give patient low-dose aspirin.
   Ask for expert help/consider thrombolysis.

This is a highly abnormal ECG for a previously fit 37-year-old woman. The ST elevation in leads I and aVL suggests an acute infarct confined to a small lateral area of the heart (the ST segment changes have not spread to the other lateral leads V5 and V6). There is reciprocal ST segment depression in the inferior leads and the anteroseptal leads. The patient should be given oxygen and intravenous pain relief. Aspirin should also be given. In view of the unusual nature of the ECG, the inpatient medical or cardiological team should be called to the department as a matter of urgency to consider further management of the patient. If the physicians are delayed then one should consider thrombolysis and ask the patient about any possible contraindications.

This woman was given 5 mg intravenous diamorphine which settled her pain. The cardiologists were called and performed an emergency coronary angiogram. This showed a single critical stenosis of the left anterior descending artery. This was successfully dilated with balloon angioplasty.

Question 11

a Raised oxygen tension with an acute respiratory alkalosis.
b Hyperventilation syndrome.

174

The blood gases show that this patient is alkalotic with a low carbon dioxide tension. A respiratory alkalosis must therefore exist. This must be acute because the base excess is within normal limits so the kidney has not yet started to compensate by retaining H^+. The perioral tingling is due to a decrease in the ionized calcium level caused by the alkalosis. In severe cases this can proceed to carpopedal spasm. Blood gases should be taken in these patients to exclude the possibility of multiple small pulmonary emboli causing hypoxia and hyperventilation.

Treatment should be aimed at reassuring the patient and slowing the respiratory rate and depth. Rebreathing using a paper bag can be tried but should not be used in patients with a history of myocardial disease.

This patient later revealed that her symptoms had developed following an attack of acute claustrophobia in the crowded supermarket.

Question 12

a Raised oxygen tension with severe metabolic acidosis and hyperventilation.

b Aspirin overdose.

c Attend to the ABCs, making sure the patient is rehydrated. Intubate the patient and perform gastric lavage.
Check urine pH. If it is not alkaline then alkalinize blood with bicarbonate.
Check blood paracetamol and salicylate levels. If salicylate levels very high, consider haemodialysis.

This patient has a severe acidosis. The large base deficit indicates that this is metabolic in origin. The patient is also hyperventilating. This may be to compensate for the metabolic acidosis or as a direct stimulant effect of salicylate on the respiratory centre. Initial asseessment should concentrate on the ABCs. A patient who is unconscious with a suspected overdose should receive a gastric lavage. She will need to have her airway protected before this procedure can be performed. Rehydration with intravenous fluids should be performed. Forced alkaline diuresis is no longer recommended because of the danger of fluid overload. It is sufficient to check that the urine pH is alkaline so that the weak salicylic acid will be excreted. If the salicylate levels are very high the patient should be considered for haemodialysis to remove the salicylate.

Question 13

a Normal Po_2 with metabolic acidosis.

b Yes. These are typical blood gases of an asthmatic who is beginning to develop respiratory failure.

c Continue patient on high flow oxygen. Call for expert help. Arrange a chest X-ray.
Repeat nebulized salbutamol 5 mg and add 500 µg ipratroprium bromide.
Give intravenous aminophylline (5 mg/kg) if the patient is not already on theophyllines; otherwise give intravenous salbutamol.
Recheck blood gases.
If patient is still deteriorating, ask anaesthetist to intubate and ventilate.

This blood gas result on first inspection does not look too severe. However a Po_2 of 12.1 kPa on high-flow oxygen is probably masking a quite severe hypoxia. The pH and base deficit show that the patient has a metabolic acidosis, probably as a combination of hypoxia and fatigue. The most worrying factor in the blood gas result is the Pco_2 of 6.4. In an asthmatic attack the Pco_2 normally falls as the patient hyperventilates. However, as the patient tires, the Pco_2 starts to rise and the patient starts to develop respiratory failure. Ventilation is necessary when the blood gases on 60% oxygen show a $Po_2 < 8$ kPa, a $Pco_2 > 6.7$ kPa or a pH < 7.2.

Question 14

a A metabolic alkalosis.

b Protracted vomiting.

The pH reveals an alkalosis. The high base excess shows that this is a metabolic alkalosis. There is some respiratory compensation with hypoventilation and a raised carbon dioxide level. Compensation does not usually return the pH to normal so the metabolic event is primary.

The most likely cause of a partially compensated metabolic alkalosis is protracted vomiting. This young girl was suffering with severe bulimia.

Question 15

a Severe hypoxia uncorrected by oxygen and combined metabolic and respiratory acidosis.

b Exacerbation of chronic obstructive airways disease with type II respiratory failure.

c Change the inspired oxygen concentration to 24% and commence a salbutamol nebulizer.

Chronic obstructive airways disease leads to alveolar hypoventilation. This leads to retention of carbon dioxide and type II ventilatory failure. These patients rely on a hypoxic respiratory drive and diminishing this with high inspired oxygen concentrations may worsen the respiratory failure. This may account for the patient's deterioration since being commenced on 60% oxygen. He should be treated with nebulized salbutamol with 24% oxygen and his gases rechecked. A search should be made for a cause of his sudden deterioration. Infection is most likely but pulmonary embolus and myocardial infarction should be excluded.

Question 16
a Pseudogout or calcium pyrophosphate arthropathy.
b Calcification of the menisci.

Pseudogout is a common age-related disease caused by deposition of calcium pyrophosphate crystals in tissues, particularly fibrocartilage. Rarely, it can be familial or associated with metabolic diseases such as Wilson's disease or hyperparathyroidism. Acute pseudogout occurs when crystals are shed from the synovial deposits. This may be precipitated by minor trauma. The crystals can be aspirated and identified under the microscope. They are small rod-shaped objects which are positively birefringent as opposed to the needle-shaped negatively birefringent crystals of acute gout.

Aspiration confirms the diagnosis and may also help symptomatology. Non-steroidal anti-inflammatory agents should also be given.

An X-ray of the knee may show calcification of the menisci. Other sites where this may be seen are the pubic symphysis and the spinal intervertebral discs.

Question 17
a No.
b No.
c Intravenous *N*-Acetylcysteine.

This patient has presented 8 hours after the overdose. This is too late to wash him out. Activated charcoal is ineffective in paracetamol overdose unless very large amounts are given. A simple rule of thumb is to give 10 times as much oral activated charcoal as the estimated amount of drug that has been taken. This patient is at risk from hepatic complications of paracetamol because of his alcoholism. The threshold line for treatment in these patients should be halved. *N*-Acetylcysteine raises intracellular levels of glutathione and mops up the toxic intermediate metabolite from the oxidation of paracetamol. He should be admitted and given a reducing dose of intravenous *N*-Acetylcysteine over the next 24 hours. His liver function should be monitored with serial measurement of his liver function tests and prothrombin time.

Question 18

a Hyperglycaemic hyperosmolar non-ketotic coma.
b Ask the physicians to admit the patient.
   Initial rehydration with normal saline.
   Insulin pump.
   Consider heparinization.

The patient is severely dehydrated with a raised blood sugar. However, he is not ketotic. A rough estimate of his blood osmolality can be made by adding twice the product of the sodium and potassium levels to his serum glucose and serum urea level. This gives a figure of 395 mosmol/kg which is grossly elevated above the normal range (275–295 mosmol/kg) and suggests the diagnosis of hyperglycaemic hyperosmolar non-ketotic coma.

This tends to occur in the elderly and is often precipitated by an underlying infection. Patients present with polyuria, polydipsia, weakness and dehydration. Treatment should commence with rehydration with normal saline and the patient should be referred to the inpatient medical team. When the severe dehydration has resolved, half-strength saline can be used. An insulin pump should be commenced but the blood sugar should not be brought down too precipitously. Potassium supplementation may also be needed. These patients are at significant risk from vascular thrombosis secondary to their sluggish circulation so heparinization should be considered. Finally the precipitating cause of the patient's deterioration should be sought.

Question 19

a Inappropriate antidiuretic hormone secretion.
b Head injury.
   Carcinoma of the bronchus.

This patient's calculated plasma osmolality is 244 mosmol/kg. He has concentrated urine. This suggests that he has inappropriate antidiuretic hormone secretion. Common causes include head injury, carcinoma of the bronchus and hypothyroidism.

Question 20

a Methanol or ethylene glycol overdose.

b Give patient alcohol to block metabolic pathway and then arrange dialysis to remove methanol or ethylene glycol.

Inspection of the electrolytes shows that the patient has an anion gap of 34 mmol/l. The bicarbonate level indicates a metabolic acidosis and the hyperventilation, that there is some respiratory compensation. Common causes of an elevated anion gap associated with a metabolic acidosis are renal failure, diabetic ketoacidosis and alcoholic ketoacidosis. However these can all be excluded in this patient with the other results. Taking note of the history the most likely cause in this patient is methanol ingestion from chronic meths drinking or ethylene glycol (antifreeze) ingestion.

Methanol or ethylene glycol poisoning should be treated by giving the patient oral alcohol. This can be in the form of several measures of spirits. This blocks the metabolic pathways of these substances. They should then be removed by haemodialysis.

CLINICAL PICTURE QUESTIONS

Clinical picture 1

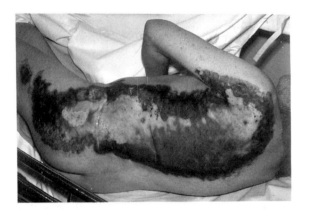

This patient fell asleep against a radiator. His back and buttock are the only areas that have been burnt.

1 What is your estimate of the size of the burn? How did you reach this figure?
2 How do you clinically determine the thickness of a burn?
3 How would you provide pain relief for this patient?

Clinical picture 2

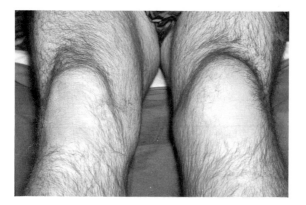

This man is a carpet-fitter. He has noticed a painful left knee for the past 2 days. On examination the knee appears as in the photograph and has a full range of movement.

1 What is the most likely diagnosis?
2 What is your treatment of this condition?
3 What other sign is present?

Clinical picture 3

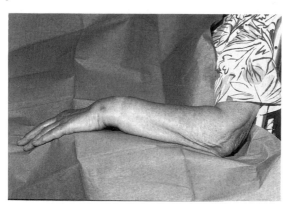

A 70-year-old woman tripped over in the street and landed on her palmar-flexed hand, sustaining the injury shown in the photograph.

1 What is the likely diagnosis?
2 How would you treat this in the A&E department?
3 What other question is it important to ask this patient?

181

Clinical picture questions

Clinical picture 4

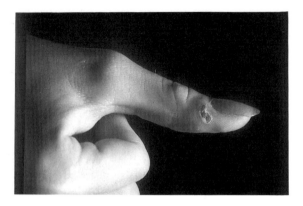

A 19-year-old nurse presents to the A&E department with this painful lesion on her finger.

1 What is the diagnosis?
2 Where else may the patient have similar lesions?
3 How would you treat this patient?

Clinical picture 5

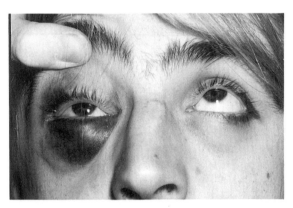

A man presents to the A&E department after being punched in the right eye.

1 What abnormal sign is being demonstrated here?
2 What other abnormal sign may you be able to elicit?
3 How would you manage this patient?

Clinical picture 6

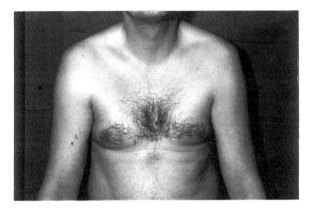

This man came to the A&E department one morning after awakening with a stiff neck and shoulders. On examination his neck movements were full but painful in all directions. He was given a soft collar and allowed home. He returned 2 days later as both of his shoulders had become very stiff.

1 What is the diagnosis?
2 How would you confirm the diagnosis?
3 How would you treat this condition?

Clinical picture 7

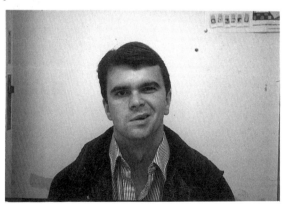

1 What is the diagnosis?
2 Of what symptoms may the patient complain?
3 What is your treatment of this patient in the A&E department?

Clinical picture questions

Clinical picture 8

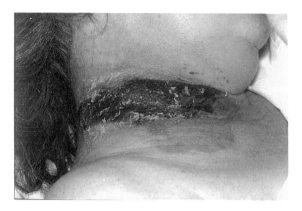

A 48-year-old alcoholic woman presented with this lesion on her neck; it had rapidly expanded over the last 48 hours.

1 What is the likely diagnosis?
2 What is the treatment of this condition?

Clinical picture 9

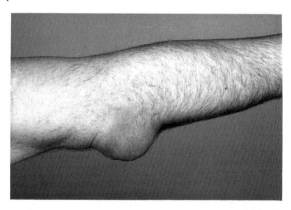

A 58-year-old man presented to the department with a painful right forefoot. He also had this lesion present on his left elbow. It was firm to touch and did not transilluminate.

1 What is the likely diagnosis?
2 Where else may the patient have a similar lesion?
3 How would you treat this patient?

Clinical picture 10

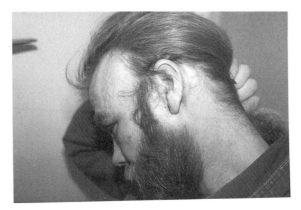

This man had presented to the department 8 hours after being assaulted.

1 What clinical sign is apparent?
2 Name three other clinical signs that may indicate the same diagnosis.

Clinical picture 11

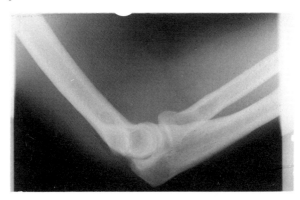

1 Name three abnormal signs visible on this X-ray.
2 How would you treat this patient?

185

Clinical picture 12

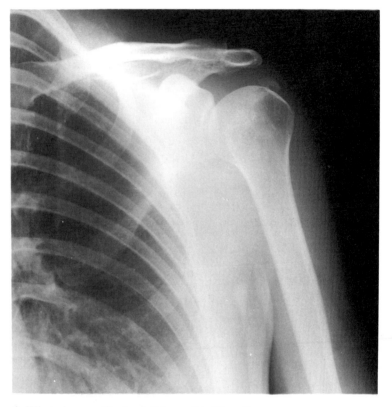

1 What abnormality is visible on this X-ray?
2 Of what symptoms may the patient complain?

Clinical picture 13

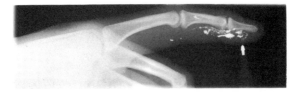

This patient was welding when he sustained this injury.

1 How would you descibe this type of injury?
2 What treatment does this patient need?

Clinical picture 14

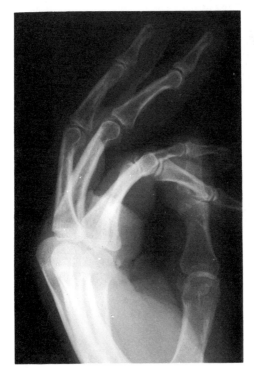

This patient has injured her left middle finger.

1 How would you describe the injury?
2 How would you suspect that the injury was caused?

Clinical picture 15

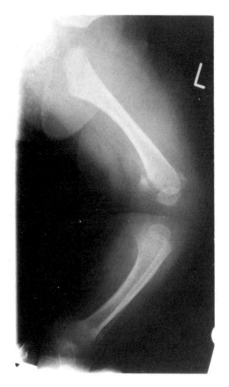

1 Describe the injury shown in this X-ray.
2 How is it likely to have been caused?

Clinical picture 16

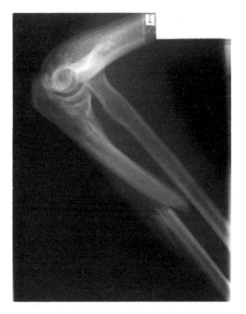

This woman fell on to her pronated hand.

1 What injuries has she sustained?
2 What is the name of this injury complex?

Clinical picture questions

Clinical picture 17

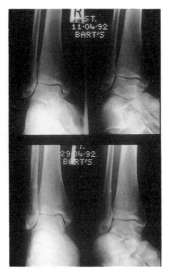

This woman came to the department complaining of a painful ankle. The X-rays are taken 2 weeks apart.

1 What is the diagnosis?
2 Name an alternative method of making the diagnosis.

Clinical picture 18

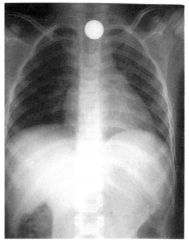

1 Where is this coin lodged?
2 What is your management of this patient?

190

Clinical picture 19

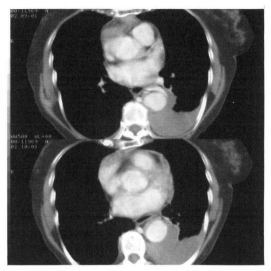

This is the chest CT scan of a 50-year-old man admitted with severe chest pain.

1 What is the diagnosis?
2 What alternative method could be used to make the diagnosis?
3 Name three factors that may predispose to this condition.

Clinical picture 20

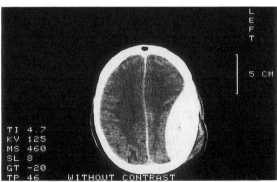

This patient had a Glasgow Coma Score of 5 prior to being intubated and this CT scan being performed.

1 Name two abnormalities visible on this CT scan.
2 How should this patient be managed?

ANSWERS TO CLINICAL PICTURE QUESTIONS

Clinical picture 1

1 Approximately 14%, determined using rule of nines.
2 Clinical appearance and sensitivity to pain.
3 Cover burns. Small amounts of IV opiates if necessary.

This alcoholic patient sustained this burn when in a drunken state. He presented to the A&E department 4 days after sustaining the injury!

Burn size should be estimated used the rule of nines (front and back of trunk each represent 18% of body surface area, the legs 18% each, the arms 9% each, the head 9% and the genitalia 1%). This rule can only be used in adults. In children the head has a relatively greater surface area. (At birth it represents 19% of the body surface area.) Estimates of smaller burns can be made using the patient's palm. This represents 1% of body surface area. The area burnt can be accurately marked on to a Lund and Browder chart.

Burns can be classified according to the thickness of tissue that has been damaged. The most superficial burns cause redness only, which resolves spontaneously within a few days. This erythema should not be measured when determining the extent of the burn.
Partial-thickness burns can be classified into superficial partial-thickness and deep dermal burns. With the former, blistering of the skin develops and the tissue looks red, angry and weepy. These burns are extremely painful. Deep dermal burns occur when most of the epidermis has been burnt away. This leaves only a few cells from which the skin can regenerate around the hair follicles and sweat glands. As the burn becomes deeper the likelihood of scarring increases. When the burn becomes full-thickness the surface takes on a dark or light, dry leathery appearance. The nerve endings have been burnt away so these burns are usually not painful.

Pain relief for patients with large burns can be accomplished in two ways. First the burn should be covered to stop circulation of air currents. This can be accomplished with Clingfilm. Second, small amounts of IV opiates should be given to the patient until the pain is controlled. This patient was not in a great deal of distress as most of the burn was full-thickness.

192

Clinical picture 2
1 Prepatellar bursitis.
2 Avoid kneeling. Use knee protection and NSAIDs.
3 Thick skin pads present over both knees.

This man has developed prepatellar bursitis or housemaid's knee. The erythema and swelling in this condition are confined to the prepatellar bursa and do not affect movement of the knee. Clergymen, who kneel with a different posture, tend to develop infrapatellar bursitis. These conditions should be treated with rest and avoidance of the precipitating factors, together with NSAIDs. Drainage of the bursa should be avoided because of the possibility of introducing pyogenic infection.

This condition is an occupational hazard for people who work kneeling down, such as cleaners, plumbers and carpet-fitters. The repetitive friction exerted on the knees in this patient is further indicated by the pads of thickened skin visible over both knees. He should be encouraged to use padded supports over his knees in the future to protect against this condition.

Clinical picture 3
1 Smith's fracture.
2 Analgesia, X-ray, then manipulate into Smith's plaster, and X-ray again for position. Refer to fracture clinic.
3 Is she right- or left-handed? What social support does the patient have at home?

The history gives to the clue to this patient's diagnosis. The forces exerted on a palmar-flexed wrist in a fall are likely to result in a fracture with volar displacement of the distal fragment. This is known as a Smith's fracture. If the picture is closely inspected it can be seen that there is no dinner-fork deformity. Instead the volar displacement of the distal fragment results in a wrist with little dorsal swelling.

These fractures should be reduced and then the patient placed in an above-elbow plaster cast with the wrist dorsiflexed and the elbow flexed to 90°. However, the fracture often redisplaces, so many authorities favour early internal fixation.

A wrist facture may have many social implications for an elderly person. Important factors to assess include whether the injury is on the dominant or non-dominant side and the level of support at home. It may be necessary to arrange for increased social service support before the patient can be safely discharged home.

Answers to clinical picture questions

Clinical picture 4
1 Herpetic paronychia.
2 Around the mouth or genitalia.
3 Topical acyclovir 5% 4-hourly.

Acute paronychia are commonly seen in A&E departments. They are usually caused by pyogenic bacteria and may be associated with biting of the nails. Early pyogenic paronychia can be treated with antibiotics, but as soon as the infection becomes localized then surgical drainage should be performed. Rarer causes of paronychia include fungal infections and the herpesvirus.

Herpetic paronychia are caused by topical spread of the herpesvirus from a cold sore or genital lesion. They can be recognized by the small vesicles present in the skin. The patient may have noticed a burning sensation prior to the development of the lesions. It is important to recognize the viral aetiology, as these patients should not be treated surgically. Instead, acyclovir 5% cream should be used. This is effective if treatment is started as soon as the first symptoms develop and is continued 4-hourly for a period of 5 days.

Clinical picture 5
1 Loss of upward gaze of the right eye secondary to tethering of he inferior rectus.
2 Infraorbital paraesthesiae.
3 X-ray to confirm diagnosis then give antibiotics and refer to ophthalmologists.

This patient is trying to look upwards. He has a blow-out fracture of the inferior orbital wall caused by a punch over the eye. Tethering of part of the inferior rectus in the fracture has resulted in loss of normal upward gaze. The inferior orbital nerve is also often damaged with this injury, resulting in paraesthesiae extending down towards the upper lip.

The diagnosis should be confirmed by X-ray. Often the fracture itself cannot be seen. However, the associated X-ray signs of a 'teardrop' seen at the superior margin of the maxillary sinus (due to the oedematous tissue bulging through the fracture) or a fluid level in the sinus, indicates the likely presence of a fracture.

The patient should be given broad-spectrum antibiotics because of the presence of an open fracture. In this case, as there is tethering of the inferior rectus, he should be referred to the ophthalmology team for further treatment. In cases where there is no ophthalmological signs, follow-up should be arranged with the maxillofacial team.

More rarely, the medial wall of the orbit may fracture, resulting in a communication with the ethmoidal sinuses. The patient may say that his eye 'bulges out' as he blows his nose. This is due to the passage of air from the sinuses into the periorbital tissues. The patient should be encouraged not to blow his nose as this may encourage the spread of pathogens into the eye.

Clinical picture 6

1 Bilateral anterior dislocations of the shoulder.
2 Arrange X-rays of the shoulders.
3 Reduce and immobilize. Refer to orthopaedic review clinic. Look for underlying causes of the event.

This man's diagnosis was initially missed. He presented complaining of pain in his neck and his shoulders but only his neck was examined. The presence of bilateral pathology where one abnormal side is similar to the other also makes the diagnosis more difficult. On reviewing the picture, the classical 'squared-off' appearance of both shoulders can be seen.

The diagnosis should be confirmed with X-ray examination. Anterior dislocation is usually apparent on an anteroposterior film but an axial view must also be taken to exclude a posterior dislocation and identify any bony fragments. If an apical film cannot be performed a lateral transthoracic view should be attempted.

Reduction of the dislocations should be performed. There are many methods of reducton. All have a failure rate and you should use the method with which you are most familiar. The arms should then be placed in slings. The patient with bilateral dislocations will have extreme difficulty in carrying out his daily activities of living without the use of his arms. He should be allowed to use his dominant arm when necessary but must be told to avoid movements that include abduction and external rotation because of the danger of recurrent dislocation. The patient should be referred for review at the next fracture clinic.

The force necessary to dislocate both shoulders is quite considerable and the event would be remembered unless the patient's level of consciousness was decreased. This can occur with an epileptic fit, although the dislocations are more frequently posterior than anterior. A history of epilepsy as a child was elucidated from this patient and he was therefore referred for medical follow-up and instructed that he should not drive.

Answers to clinical picture questions

Clinical picture 7
1 Right facial palsy (lower motor neuron).
2 Unilateral weakness of facial muscles. Pain behind the mastoid, hyperacusis, welling of tears in the eye and an altered sensation of taste.
3 Exclude obvious causes of facial palsy. Ask GP to refer patient to neurology outpatient department for follow-up.

This patient presented to the department with a 1-day history of facial weakness. On examination the palsy can be seen to be lower motor neuron in nature because of loss of use of the forehead muscles. If no cause can be found for this lesion then it can be termed a Bell's palsy.

As the seventh cranial nerve gives motor innervation to the facial muscles and stapedius, secretory innervation to the lacrimal gland and taste innervation to the anterior two-thirds of the tongue, a palsy may produce a wide spectrum of symptomatology.

The role of the A&E physician should be to ensure that the palsy is peripheral in nature and to exclude any other neurological involvement. The corneal reflex should be intact and the adjacent cranial nerves V, VI and VIII should be tested. The eardrum and the parotid gland must also be inspected to exclude any local causes of facial palsy. If no other abnormalities can be found, a provisional diagnosis of Bell's palsy can be made. Follow-up should be arranged via the GP. Most patients attain complete or near-complete recovery within 2 weeks to 2 months. Some experts advocate the usage of steroids in the acute phase but this will vary according to local policy.

Clinical picture 8
1 Necrotizing fasciitis.
2 Fluid resuscitation. Swab and commence intravenous broad-spectrum antibiotics; refer to surgical team for debridement of wound.

Necrotizing fasciitis is a rapidly spreading infection of the skin, subcutaneous tissue and fascia. Diabetes, alcoholism, peripheral vascular disease and trauma are predisposing factors.

In 1994 many reports of the condition were publicized in the news headlines with titles such as 'the flesh-eating virus'. The disease incidence has actually remained constant over the years and it is caused by a number of bacteria rather than by a virus. Gram-positive cocci such as *Streptococcus* and *Staphylococcus*, Gram-negative bacilli such as *Enterobacter* and *Pseudomonas* and anaerobes are the usual infecting organisms.

The treatment of necrotizing fasciitis should start with fluid resuscitation, intravenous broad-spectrum antibiotics according to the likely pathogens, early and extensive surgical incision and drainage with debridement. The large volumes of fluid lost into the wound, coupled with systemic toxicity and DIC, result in a mortality rate of 20–50%.

Clinical picture 9
1 Acute gout with gouty tophus on elbow.
2 Forearms, hands, knees, Achilles tendon, feet, helix of the ear.
3 With an NSAID.

The presence of a lesion on the elbow and a tender forefoot point to the diagnosis of gout. Uric acid crystals are deposited from supersaturated extracellular fluid into joint spaces, producing gouty arthritis, and into musculotendinous units, producing tophi. The most common joints to be affected are the hallux metatarsophalangeal joint, the tarsal joints, the ankle and the knee. Tophi are commonly seen in the olecranon bursa, over the ulnar surface of the arms, in the helix of the ears and in knees, feet and toes.

Diagnosis in the A&E department is usually clinical. A serum uric acid is not helpful in the acute attack and may be normal. Important differential diagnoses such as septic arthritis should be excluded and the patient's renal function should be checked. X-rays may be of help if the condition is more chronic, showing asymmetrical bone erosions. A definitive diagnosis can be made if a joint aspirate is examined under polarized light for negatively birefringent urate crystals.

Treatment of the acute attack should commence with an NSAID such as ibuprofen. If the patient is unable to tolerate NSAIDs, colchicine can be used. Long-term therapy with a uricosuric drug such as allopurinol should not be commenced with the acute episode as it may worsen symptomatology.

Clinical picture 10
1 Battle's sign.
2 Raccoon eyes, haemotympanum, cerebrospinal fluid, rhinorrhoea or otorrhoea.

Bruising over the mastoid process is a sign of a basilar skull fracture. Other clinical signs include haemotympanum or cerebrospinal fluid otorrhoea if the fracture extends through the middle ear and

197

cerebrospinal fluid rhinorrhoea if the fracture has passed through the cribriform plate. The diagnosis is usually clinical as radiological abnormalities are rare. Occasionally a blood–air fluid level will be seen on the skull X-ray as an indirect sign of a basal fracture.

These patients should be admitted overnight for observation because of the increased association of intracranial haemorrhage associated with skull fracture. The other potential complications are a persistent cerebrospinal fluid leak and intracranial infection. Cerebrospinal fluid leaks usually repair spontaneously within 2 weeks. Otherwise, surgical repair needs to be undertaken. Most authorities give these patients a course of prophylactic antibiotics whilst the leak exists, although there is little evidence that this is of benefit.

Clinical picture 11
1 Fractured radial head, raised anterior fat pad, posterior fat pad.
2 Aspirate haemarthrosis and inject local anaesthetic, apply a broad arm sling and arrange review in fracture clinic.

This film indicates the importance of looking at the soft tissues as well as looking at bones when inspecting an X-ray. Often the only sign of a radial head injury will be the presence of abnormal fat pads. On a normal lateral X-ray of the elbow, a narrow strip of radiolucency anterior to the lower humerus is present as an anterior fat pad. Posteriorly the fat is hidden in the concavity of the coronoid and olecranon fossa and cannot be seen. If there is a fracture

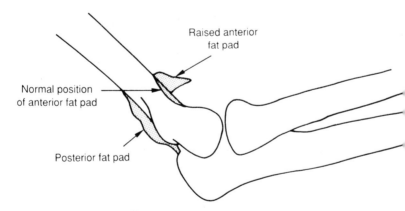

Fig. 3 Fracture producing intra-articular haemorrhage causes blood to distend the synovial capsule, displacing the fat out of the fossae, producing a visible posterior fat pad and raising the anterior fat pad.

producing intra-articular haemorrhage, the blood distends the synovial capsule, displacing the fat out of the fossae, producing a visible posterior fat pad and raising the anterior fat pad so that it looks like a ship's pennant (Fig. 3).

These fractures can be divided into three groups. Type I, as in this patient, are undisplaced fractures. Type II are displaced marginal fractures and type III are comminuted fractures. Type I fractures are treated with aspiration of the haemarthrosis and injection of local anaesthetic. This produces marked symptomatic relief. They should then be placed in a broad arm sling and follow-up arranged in the fracture clinic. If pain is severe, a back-slab can be applied. Mobilization after 2–3 weeks is encouraged. Type II fractures should be treated with more prolonged immobilization, followed by slowly increasing mobility exercises. If the fracture is comminuted, radial head excision is usually necessary to regain a good range of movement at the elbow.

Clinical picture 12
1 Calcification in the supraspinatus tendon.
2 'Painful arc' syndrome or total loss of arm abduction.

Supraspinous tendinitis results from overuse of the upper limb, which causes repetitive small strains of the tendon fibres. With time, calcification of the tendon occurs. The patient usually complains of pain when the arm is abducted to 60° or greater – the so-called 'painful arc'. At this point the tendon impinges beneath the acromion and friction occurs.

Treatment should consist of rest from the provoking activities and a course of NSAIDs. Complete rest for greater than 2 days should be avoided because of the risk of developing adhesive capsulitis at the shoulder. Injection of a local steroid may help but this should be arranged by the physician who is going to assume long-term care for the patient.

Clinical picture 13
1 High-pressure injection injury.
2 Tetanus prophylaxis, prophylactic antibiotics and urgent operative debridement.

This injury was sustained when a molten metal splinter penetrated the middle finger of this welder's left hand. The metal has solidified, outlining the flexor tendon sheath. This is an unusual example of a high-pressure injection wound. These are serious injuries caused by the injection of liquid at high pressure and speed into the tissues of the hand. More common causes are grease and paint guns. The entry wound may be very small and the patient may initially only notice mild swelling and paraesthesia of the affected area. However, the foreign material will have spread widely across the fascial planes and rapidly causes a severe inflammatory response.

The diagnosis should be suspected on the history and the patient referred for urgent debridement. Tetanus cover and broad-spectrum antibiotics should be given. Surgical outcome is reasonable after injection with hydraulic fluids but amputation is often necessary with more irritant substances such as paint or molten metal.

Clinical picture 14

1 Volar plate avulsion fracture of proximal interphalangeal joint of the left middle finger.
2 Hyperextension injury.

A fibrocartilaginous volar plate provides volar support for the proximal interphalangeal joints of the fingers. In hyperextension injuries this plate can be torn off, together with a small fragment of bone. An avulsion fragment is also often seen with a dorsal dislocation at the proximal interphalangeal joint.

The finger should be examined to ensure that the radial and ulnar collateral ligaments are intact. If one of these ligaments is partially torn the joint will be stable but there will be tenderness over the affected area. If the tear is complete, the joint will open out during stress testing. When stable, the finger can be treated with buddy strapping and early mobilization. If unstable, expert advice should be sought. All proximal interphalangeal joint injuries should be followed up in a hand clinic because of the high degree of associated morbidity.

This woman sustained her injury when her fingers were hyperextended catching a basketball.

Clinical picture 15

1 Metaphyseal 'corner' fractures of distal femur (Salter-Harris II).
2 Non-accidental injury by twisting the infant's leg.

Skeletal injuries in an unusual site in a child should alert the physician to the possibility of non-accidental injury. The most characteristic injuries are separation of the epiphyses or metaphyseal chip or corner fractures. These are caused by grasping and twisting forces applied to the affected limb. Other fractures that occur more commonly in non-accidental injury but are less pathognomonic are transverse and spiral fractures of long bones, skull fractures and multiple paravertebral rib fractures.

If the diagnosis of non-accidental injury is suspected, senior paediatric help should be requested and the social work team informed. It is usually best to leave further investigation of these children and families to the paediatricians because of the complex issues that are involved and the ongoing nature of care that will be needed.

Clinical picture 16
1 Dislocated radial head and fractured midshaft of ulnar.
2 Monteggia fracture dislocation.

In the forearm, injury to one bone usually leads to fracture or dislocation of the other. The exception is the 'nightstick' fracture caused by a direct blow. All injuries to the forearm should have the full length of both bones X-rayed in two planes.

This woman was referred to the orthopaedic team for reduction and internal fixation of her injury.

Clinical picture 17
1 Stress fracture of the right fibula.
2 Radioisotope scanning.

On some occasions bony injuries cannot be visualized on X-rays. One such instance occurs when there is a stress fracture. These are common in the metatarsals of the feet, the 'march' fracture, but may also develop in other bones such as the fibula or femoral neck. The diagnosis can be made by X-raying the patient at a later date when callus will have developed around the fracture or by arranging a bone scan of the affected area. Increased osteoblastic and osteoclastic activity will then reveal the fracture.

Impacted fractures of the femur can also be very difficult to see on X-ray and are frequently missed. In general, if the patient is symptomatic of a fracture, rely on clinical findings and treat as appropriate for that injury.

Clinical picture 18
1 In the upper oesophagus in the postcricoid area.
2 Removal of the coin using an oesophagoscope.

Young children frequently swallow small objects such as button batteries, peanuts and coins. They should be examined closely to see if there is any evidence that the foreign body has passed into the lungs. An X-ray must always be taken to ensure that the foreign body is not lodging in a bronchus causing lung collapse or has not lodged in the oesophagus. Delay in diagnosis may lead to oesophageal erosion with subsequent perforation or stricture formation. Smooth objects tend to obstruct the oesophagus in three areas – in the postcricoid area, at the level of the aortic arch and at the gastro-oesophageal junction.

The coin should be removed using an oesophagoscope under a general anaesthetic. If it passes into the stomach it is likely to pass through the rest of the gastrointestinal tract without complication. The parents should be asked to check the child's faeces and return in 3 days if the coin has not passed.

Clinical picture 19
1 Aortic dissection.
2 By arch aortography.
3 Cystic medial necrosis.
   Trauma.
   Atheroma.

This CT scan shows the intimal flap of an aortic dissection, dividing the aorta into a true and false lumen. The appearance is known as the 'tennis ball' sign. Diagnosis of aortic dissection can be made by CT scan but arteriography (an arch aortogram) is preferred, as it is more reliable and gives more anatomical detail.

Aortic dissection occurs in three groups of people. It can develop as a result of a congenital weakness of the aortic wall, known as cystic medial necrosis (seen in patients with Marfan's syndrome and those with pseudoxanthoma elasticum). It also occurs as a result of atheroma and finally may be seen in trauma patients, particularly in those where large decelerative forces have been involved.

Clinical picture 20
1 Acute left-sided extradural haemorrhage.
   Mass effect with midline shift of ventricle.
2 Urgent evacuation of extradural blood.

This patient has an acute extradural haemorrhage with mass effect causing midline shift and compression of the right ventricle. An extradural haemorrhage is caused by an arterial bleed and strips off the dura from the inner table of the skull, resulting in a biconvex or lens-like appearance. This differentiates it from the venous subdural bleed which spreads around over the surface of the brain, giving a half-moon appearance.

Management must be aimed at removing the blood as soon as possible. A neurosurgeon should be contacted. He or she may advise using mannitol to try and reduce intracranial pressure whilst the patient is being taken to theatre. Other measures that should be taken to keep the intracranial pressure as low as possible are hyperventilation (which reduces the arterial carbon dioxide) and nursing the patient tilted head-up.

RECOMMENDED READING

Advanced Life Support Group (1993) *Advanced Paediatric Life Support*. BMJ Publications

American College of Surgeons (1993) *Advanced Trauma Life Support Course Programme*

Apley and Soloman (1991) *Concise System of Orthopaedics and Trauma*. Butterworth-Heinemann

Collier, Longmore and Harvey (1994) *Oxford Handbook of Clinical Specialities,* 3rd edn. Oxford Medical Publications

Eaton (1992) *Essentials of Immediate Medical Care*. Churchill Livingstone

Forbes and Jackson (1993) *A Colour Atlas and Text of Clinical Medicine*. Wolfe

Greaves, Porter and Dyer (eds) (1995) *A Handbook of Immediate Medical Care*. Ballière Tindall

Hall and Johnson (1993) *Essential Paediatrics*. Churchill Livingstone

Johnson and Fosarelli (1993) *Paediatric Pearls,* 2nd edn. Mosby

Kumar and Clarke (1990) *Clinical Medicine,* 2nd edn. Ballière Tindall

Lindsay, Bone and Callander (1986) *Neurology and Neurosurgery Illustrated*. Churchill Livingstone

McRae (1989) *Practical Fracture Management,* 3rd edn. Churchill Livingstone

Morton and Phillips (1992) *Accidents and Emergencies in Children*. Oxford University Press

Proudfoot (1994) *Acute Poisoning*. Butterworth-Heinemann

Robertson and Redmond (1991) *The Management of Major Trauma*. Oxford University Press

Weatherall, Ledingham and Warrell (eds) (1987) *Oxford Textbook of Medicine,* 2nd edn. Oxford University Press.

Yates and Redmond (1985) *Lecture Notes on Accident and Emergency Medicine*. Blackwell Scientific Publications

Index

Index

Index

Index

Index

Index

Index

Index

Index